ADOLESCENT MEDICINE CLINICS

Contraception and Adolescents

GUEST EDITORS
Robert T. Brown, MD
Paula K. Braverman, MD

October 2005 • Volume 16 • Number 3

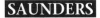

An Imprint of Elsevier, Inc.
PHILADELPHIA   LONDON   TORONTO   MONTREAL   SYDNEY   TOKYO

W.B. SAUNDERS COMPANY
A Division of Elsevier Inc.

1600 John F. Kennedy Blvd., Suite 1800, Philadelphia, PA 19103-2899

http://www.theclinics.com

Learning Resources
Centre

12972444

ADOLESCENT MEDICINE CLINICS
October 2005
Editor: Carin Davis

Volume 16, Number 3
ISSN 1547-3368
ISBN 1-4160-2645-2

Reprints. For copies of 100 or more of articles in this publication, please contact the Commercial Reprints Department, Elsevier Inc., 360 Park Avenue South, New York, New York 10010-1710. Tel.: (212) 633-3818, Fax: (212) 462-1935, email: reprints@elsevier.com

The ideas and opinions expressed in *Adolescent Medicine Clinics* do not necessarily reflect those of the Publisher. The Publisher does not assume any responsibility for any injury and/or damage to persons or property arising out of or related to any use of the material contained in this periodical. The reader is advised to check the appropriate medical literature and the product information currently provided by the manufacturer of each drug to be administered toverify the dosage, the method and duration of administration, or contraindications. It is the responsibility of the treating physician or other health care professional, relying on independent experience and knowledge of the patient, to determine drug dosages and the best treatment for the patient. Mention of any product in this issue should not be construed as endorsement by the contributors, editors, or the Publisher of the product or manufacturers' claims.

Adolescent Medicine Clinics (ISSN 1547-3368) is published in February, June, and October by Elsevier. Corporate and editorial offices: 1600 John F. Kennedy Blvd., Suite 1800, Philadelphia, PA 19103-2899. Accounting and circulation offices: 6277 Sea Harbor Drive, Orlando, FL 32887-4800. Subscription prices are $95.00 per year for US individuals, $133.00 per year for US institutions, $48.00 per year for US students, $150.00 per year for Canadian institutions, $53.00 per year for Canadian students. To receive student/resident rate, orders must be accompanied by name of affiliated institution, date of term, and the signature of program/residency coordinator on institution letterhead. Orders will be billed at individual rate until proof of status is received. Foreign air speed delivery is included in all Clinics subscription prices. All prices are subject to change without notice. POSTMASTER: Send address changes to *Adolescent Medicine Clinics,* W.B. Saunders Company, Periodicals Fulfillment, Orlando, FL 32887-4800. **Customer Service: 1-800-654-2452 (US). From outside of the US, call 1-407-345-4000.**

Adolescent Medicine Clinics is covered in *Index Medicus/MEDLINE,* the *Combined Cumulative Index to Pediatrics,* ISI/ISTP & B online database, Index to Scientific Book Contents, Biological Abstracts/RRM, and Current Contents (Clinical Medicine and Social & Behavioral Sciences).

Printed in the United States of America.

Adolescent Medicine Clinics

Official Journal of the
Section on Adolescent Health of the American Academy of Pediatrics

EDITORS-IN-CHIEF

VICTOR C. STRASBURGER, MD, Professor, Departments of Pediatrics and Family and Community Medicine; Chief, Division of Adolescent Medicine, University of New Mexico School of Medicine, Albuquerque, New Mexico

DONALD E. GREYDANUS, MD, Professor, Pediatrics and Human Development, Michigan State University College of Human Medicine; and Director, Pediatrics Program, Michigan State University Kalamazoo Center for Medical Studies, Kalamazoo, Michigan

GUEST EDITORS

ROBERT T. BROWN, MD, Professor, Section of Adolescent Health, Department of Pediatrics, Children's Hospital, The Ohio State University College of Medicine, Columbus, Ohio

PAULA K. BRAVERMAN, MD, Professor, Clinical Pediatrics, University of Cincinnati College of Medicine; Division of Adolescent Medicine, Department of Pediatrics, Cincinnati Children's Hospital Medical Center, Cincinnati, Ohio

CONTRIBUTORS

EMMA ALESNA-LLANTO, MD, FPPS, Clinical Associate Professor, Department of Pediatrics, College of Medicine–Philippine General Hospital, University of the Philippines Manila, Manila, Philippines

ANDREA E. BONNY, MD, Assistant Professor of Pediatrics, Case Western Reserve University School of Medicine; Division of Adolescent Medicine, MetroHealth Medical Center, Cleveland, Ohio

CORA COLLETTE BREUNER, MD, MPH, Associate Professor, Adolescent Medicine Section, Department of Pediatrics, Children's Hospital and Medical Center, Seattle, Washington

AMY M. BURKETT, MD, Clinical Instructor, Department of Obstetrics and Gynecology, The Ohio State University College of Medicine and School of Public Health, Columbus, Ohio

MICHELE E. CALDERONI, DO, Assistant Professor of Pediatrics and Medicine, Section of Adolescent Medicine, Children's Hospital at Montefiore/Albert Einstein College of Medicine, Bronx, New York

LEE ANN E. CONARD, RPh, DO, MPH, Assistant Professor of Pediatrics, Division of Adolescent Medicine, University of Pittsburgh School of Medicine, Children's Hospital of Pittsburgh, Pittsburgh, Pennsylvania

SUSAN COUPEY, MD, Professor of Pediatrics, Section Chief, Adolescent Medicine, Children's Hospital at Montefiore/Albert Einstein College of Medicine, Bronx, New York

BARBARA A. CROMER, MD, Professor of Pediatrics, Case Western University School of Medicine; Director, Division of Adolescent Medicine, MetroHealth Medical Center, Cleveland, Ohio

BLANCA C. DE GUIA, MD, MSc, Associate Professor of Obstetrics and Gynecology, University of the Philippines College of Medicine and Philippine General Hospital, Manila, Philippines

ELISSA B. GITTES, MD, Assistant Professor, University of Missouri-Kansas City School of Medicine; Children's Mercy Hospital and Clinics, Section of Developmental and Behavioral Sciences, Kansas City, Missouri

MELANIE A. GOLD, DO, Associate Professor of Pediatrics, Division of Adolescent Medicine, University of Pittsburgh School of Medicine, Children's Hospital of Pittsburgh, Pittsburgh, Pennsylvania

LAURA S. HARKNESS, PhD, Assistant Professor of Pediatrics and Nutrition, Case Western Reserve University School of Medicine; Division of Adolescent Medicine, MetroHealth Medical Center, Cleveland, Ohio

GERI D. HEWITT, MD, Associate Clinical Professor of Obstetrics and Gynecology and Pediatrics, The Ohio State University College of Medicine and School of Public Health, Columbus, Ohio

PAULA J. ADAMS HILLARD, MD, Professor of Obstetrics and Gynecology, Professor of Pediatrics, University of Cincinnati College of Medicine, Cincinnati, Ohio

MARY ANNE JAMIESON, MD, FRCSC, Associate Professor and Director of Pediatric and Adolescent Gynecology, Department of Obstetrics and Gynecology, Queen's University, Kingston, Ontario, Canada

JENNA McNAUGHT, MD, FRCSC, Contraceptive Advice, Research and Education (C.A.R.E.) Fellow, Department of Obstetrics and Gynecology, Queen's University, Kingston, Ontario, Canada

KRISTI MORGAN MULCHAHEY, MD, Atlanta Gynecology Associates, Marietta, Georgia

HATIM A. OMAR, MD, Professor of Pediatrics and Obstetrics and Gynecology, Section of Adolescent Medicine, University of Kentucky College of Medicine, Lexington, Kentucky

KRISTIN M. RAGER, MD, MPH, Assistant Professor of Pediatrics, Section of Adolescent Medicine, University of Kentucky College of Medicine, Lexington, Kentucky

CORAZON M. RAYMUNDO, MA, MS, DSc, Professor of Demography–Population Institute, University of the Philippines Diliman, Quezon City, Philippines

KATHLEEN Z. REAPE, MD, FACOG, Director, Clinical Operations, Duramed Research, Inc., Bala Cynwyd, Pennsylvania

JULIE L. STRICKLAND, MD, MPH, Associate Professor, Department of Obstetrics and Gynecology, University of Missouri-Kansas City School of Medicine, Kansas City, Missouri; Division of Gynecology, Children's Mercy Hospital, Overland Park, Kansas

CONTENTS

Preface xv
Robert T. Brown and Paula K. Braverman

Overview of Contraception 485
Paula J. Adams Hillard

> The United States has the highest rates of adolescent pregnancy of
> any Western industrialized country. Addressing these high rates and
> preventing adolescent pregnancy are complicated tasks. This article
> addresses some of the issues involved with preventing adolescent
> pregnancy, focusing on contraception.

Barrier and Spermicidal Contraceptives in Adolescence 495
Jenna McNaught and Mary Anne Jamieson

> This article describes both barrier and spermicide methods of
> contraception including the male and female condom, diaphragm,
> contraceptive sponge, Lea Shield, cervical cap and multiple sper-
> micide options. Their efficacy, differences and proper use are dis-
> cussed with an emphasis on the adolescent user.

Combined Hormonal Contraception 517
Michele E. Calderoni and Susan M. Coupey

> This article discusses the different combined hormonal contracep-
> tion methods. Combined methods, delivering both estrogen and a
> progestin simultaneously, are among the most effective, widely
> used hormonal contraceptive options. They also have the best non-
> contraceptive benefit profile for young women of all hormonal
> contraceptive options. Oral contraceptive pills (OCPs) are described
> as the standard combined hormonal method and are discussed in
> detail. Newer combined hormonal contraceptive delivery systems,
> the transdermal patch, vaginal ring, and injectable form, are com-
> pared with OCPs in terms of pharmacology, efficacy, and adverse

events. Advantages and disadvantages of all methods are empha-sized, with particular attention to adolescent development and acceptability.

Hormonal Contraception: Noncontraceptive Benefits and Medical Contraindications 539
Kristin M. Rager and Hatim A. Omar

This article delineates the noncontraceptive benefits of hormonal contraception, including combined and progestin-only methods. Contraindications to the use of these hormonal methods also are discussed. Knowledge of the noncontraceptive benefits of birth control methods can increase compliance and continuation of use, with the ultimate goal of decreasing unplanned pregnancy.

Progestin Only Contraceptives and Their Use in Adolescents: Clinical Options and Medical Indications 553
Amy M. Burkett and Geri D. Hewitt

Some adolescents use progestin only contraceptive products because of an underlying medical condition; others simply prefer them. Current options include pills, a long-acting intramuscular injection, an implant, and a progestin-releasing intrauterine device. Also avail-able is Plan B, a progestin only emergency contraceptive option. Although these products vary in efficacy, they are generally safe and well tolerated by adolescents. The implants and intramuscular injections are particularly well suited for adolescent use because of their need for little compliance, well-tolerated adverse effect profile, and excellent efficacy rates.

Depot Medroxyprogesterone Acetate: Implications for Weight Status and Bone Mineral Density in the Adolescent Female 569
Andrea E. Bonny, Laura S. Harkness, and Barbara A. Cromer

Depot medroxyprogesterone acetate (DMPA) is an effective and easy-to-use contraceptive method for adolescents. However, recent literature suggests that overweight teens may be at increased risk for weight gain while on this contraceptive method, and decreases in bone mineral density have been documented in adolescents on DMPA, particularly with longer duration of use. Consideration of this new literature on DMPA and its implications for clinical prac-tice must be done in the context of the United States having the highest adolescent pregnancy rate in the industrialized world. Hence, potential DMPA risks need to be weighed against the risk of unintended pregnancy in an adolescent.

Emergency Contraception   585

Lee Ann E. Conard and Melanie A. Gold

Emergency contraception is increasing in use and has become a
universal standard of care in the United States. This article reviews
available forms of emergency contraception, their indications, contraindications, adverse effects and efficacy at preventing pregnancy.
This article describes the mechanism of action of different forms of
emergency contraception and provides recommendations on when
to start or restart an ongoing method of contraception after emergency contraception use. Literature on the impact of the advance
provision of emergency contraception on contracepting behaviors
is reviewed, and behavior change counseling related to emergency
contraception is described.

Natural Contraception   603

Cora Collette Breuner

This article discusses some complementary and alternative medicine options for contraception, including natural family planning
and plant-derived hormonal contraception. Primary care providers
are crucial resources for advice and recommendations about these
options. The discussion will include medical evidence to support
or refute these methods, potential dangers of these interventions,
and additional resources for those who want to learn more.

Current Contraceptive Research and Development   617

Kathleen Z. Reape

The approval of various new contraceptive products in recent years
has resulted in broadening the options available to women. Trends
in contraceptive research for hormonal products include variations in
dose and dosing regimens, introduction of novel compounds, evaluation of products for noncontraceptive indications, and development
of nonoral delivery systems and male contraceptives. Nonhormonal
areas of research include microbicidal products, dual protection
methods, and contraceptive vaccines. For each of these categories,
contraceptive products currently in development and the potential
implications for adolescents are discussed. Ongoing contraceptive
research and development activity is robust and should ensure the
continued availability of various new products for adolescents.

Contraceptive Choices for Chronically Ill Adolescents   635

Elissa B. Gittes and Julie L. Strickland

Ten percent of teenagers have chronic medical illness and need effective contraception for pregnancy prevention. There are available
safe and effective methods; however, the selection of a contraceptive
may be challenging because of the complexity of the underlying

medical illness. This article offers options for contraception for girls with various chronic medical conditions. Considerations of some of the newer contraception methods are discussed as future options for these girls.

Contraceptive Issues of Youth and Adolescents in Developing Countries: Highlights from the Philippines and Other Asian Countries   645
Emma Alesna-Llanto and Corazon M. Raymundo

This article highlights the contraceptive issues in Asia, home to some 700 million adolescents. It starts with a description of the socio-cultural milieu of adolescents in South and Southeast Asia, their knowledge and use of contraceptives, the myriad barriers to access, and the many innovative programs to broaden contraceptive availability. The reproductive health needs of adolescents in poor countries cannot be solved by merely supplying them with contraceptives—these needs can only be fully addressed in the context of gender equality, poverty alleviation and the conviction that investing in reproductive health of adolescents is a most urgent priority. Investing in the reproductive health of adolescents will have an impact not only on birth and abortion rates, maternal health, and the spread of STI/HIV but also on the demographics and economic development of the region—and beyond.

Practical Approaches to Prescribing Contraception in the Office Setting   665
Kristi Morgan Mulchahey

Caring for the contraceptive needs of an adolescent young woman can be a challenge on many levels. Adolescents are often called young adults, but they are not adults developmentally. Therefore, adult strategies for contraceptive teaching, decision making, and compliance are often inappropriate and unsuccessful. Health care providers are faced with increasing constraints in the office that can make it difficult to find the time to counsel the adolescent appropriately. Parental involvement in contraceptive decision making, compliance, and continuation will be different with each adolescent and her family. Although this interaction can be a problem, it is also an area where the clinician may make a positive impact for the adolescent and her family.

Erratum   675
Sarah L. Ashby and Michael Rich

Cumulative Index 2005   677

FORTHCOMING ISSUES

February 2006

Psychiatry and Behavioral Problems
Richard E. Kriepe, MD, and
Christopher Hodgman, MD, *Guest Editors*

June 2006

Substance Abuse
Manuel Schydlower, MD, and
Rodolofo Arredondo, EdD, *Guest Editors*

October 2006

Hot Topics in Adolescent Medicine
John Kulig, MD, MPH, and
Rebecca O'Brien, MD, *Guest Editors*

RECENT ISSUES

June 2005

Adolescents and the Media
Victor C. Strasburger, MD, and
Marjorie J. Hogan, MD, *Guest Editors*

February 2005

Nephrologic Disorders in the Adolescent
Jules Sherwinter, MD,
D. Michael Foulds, MD, and
Donald E. Greydanus, MD, *Guest Editors*

October 2004

Surgical Issues in Adolescents
Marjorie J. Arca, MD, and
Geri Hewitt, MD, *Guest Editors*

The Clinics are now available online!

http://www.theclinics.com

ELSEVIER
SAUNDERS

Adolesc Med 16 (2005) xv–xvi

ADOLESCENT
MEDICINE
CLINICS

Preface

Contraception and Adolescents

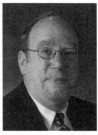 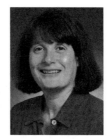

Robert T. Brown, MD   Paula K. Braverman, MD
Guest Editors

Although everyone acknowledges that the best contraception for adolescents is abstinence, many young people choose to become sexually active. Providing them with the most up-to-date information and guidance is crucial in helping to prevent the negative consequences of their sexual activity (eg, pregnancy and sexually transmitted infections). This issue of the *Adolescent Medicine Clinics* offers the latest information on all aspects of contraception for adolescents. Each article contains the most recent information from experts in the field to help clinicians guide young patients in discussions about this very important area of adolescent health.

The editors wish to thank the contributors for their excellent work preparing these articles. Special comment should be made about the need for information about contraception for young people throughout the world; the article on contraception in developing countries is particularly pertinent in that regard. It is our hope that clinicians everywhere will find this issue of the *Adolescent Medicine Clinics* useful for many years to come.

1547-3368/05/$ – see front matter © 2005 Elsevier Inc. All rights reserved.
doi:10.1016/j.admecli.2005.07.001   *adolescent.theclinics.com*

Robert T. Brown, MD
Section of Adolescent Health
Children's Hospital
Department of Pediatrics
The Ohio State University
College of Medicine
700 Children's Drive
Columbus, OH 43205-2696, USA
E-mail address: brownr@pediatrics.ohio-state.edu

Paula K. Braverman, MD
Division of Adolescent Medicine
Department of Pediatrics
Cincinnati Children's Hospital Medical Center
University of Cincinnati College of Medicine
Mail Location 4000 3333 Burnet Avenue
Cincinnati, OH 45229, USA
E-mail address: paula.braverman@cchmc.org

ELSEVIER
SAUNDERS

Adolesc Med 16 (2005) 485–493

Overview of Contraception

Paula J. Adams Hillard, MD*

University of Cincinnati College of Medicine, Cincinnati, OH, USA

The United States has the highest rates of adolescent pregnancy and birth of any country in the industrialized Western world; adolescent pregnancy rates in the United States are more than two to three times the rates of Canada or Europe and eight times higher than rates in the Netherlands and Japan [1]. It has been estimated that approximately one third of American girls will experience at least one pregnancy before the age of 20, even taking into account declining adolescent pregnancy rates from the early 1990s to 2002 [2]. Approximately 820,000 adolescent pregnancies occurred in the United States in 2003 [3]. The rate of adolescent births in the United States has fallen since its high in the early 1950s and since a recent peak in the 1990s to a new low of 41.7 births per 1000 adolescents aged 15 to 19 years; this represents a 33% drop since 1991 [4] (Fig. 1). The rate for 10- to 14-year-olds has declined by 57% [4] (Fig. 2). Depending on how the question is phrased and when it is asked, 70% to 90% of adolescent pregnancies are unplanned [5,6]. In the latest year for which statistics are available, 2000, 57% of adolescent pregnancies ended in birth; approximately 14% end in spontaneous abortion, and 29% end in abortion [3]. When contraception fails, adolescents may elect to terminate their pregnancies. Abortion rates impact adolescent birth rates, and abortion rates for adolescents fell during the 1990s [12] (Fig. 3). The abortion ratio—the ratio of abortions to live births—is higher among adolescents than older women, and is highest among those younger than 15 [12].

Few adolescent pregnancies result in infants being placed for adoption; less than 1% of teens chose to place their children for adoption in a 1995 survey [7].

* Cincinnati Children's Hospital Medical Center, Division of Adolescent Medicine, 3333 Burnet Avenue, ML 4000, Cincinnati, OH 45229.

E-mail address: paula.hillard@cchmc.org

1547-3368/05/$ – see front matter © 2005 Elsevier Inc. All rights reserved.
doi:10.1016/j.admecli.2005.05.008 *adolescent.theclinics.com*

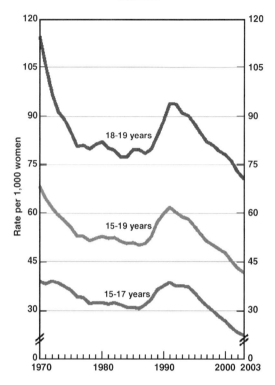

Fig. 1. Birth rates for teenagers by age: United States, 1970 to 2003, National Vital Statistics Reports, Vol. 53, No. 9, November 23, 2004.

This percentage represents a sharp decline since the 1940s. Fewer black women and teens placed a child for adoption than did white women and teens [8].

The percentage of adolescents who were sexually active increased from the early 1970s through the late 1980s, and the overall teen pregnancy rate must be interpreted in this context [9]. In 1970, the first year of the National Surveys of Family Growth (NSFG), fewer than 50% of 19-year-olds had had sexual intercourse. By the mid-1980s, more than 50% of 17-year-olds were sexually experienced. Since that time, it appears that rates of sexual activity have plateaued [10]. It has been estimated, that the sharp decline in adolescent pregnancy rates, in spite of stable rates of sexual activity, is due in part to more effective contraceptive use. Darroch has estimated that 75% of the decline in adolescent pregnancy rates is due to more effective contraception, whereas 25% is due to an increasing focus on and choice of abstinence [10]. Santelli estimated that improved contraceptive practice and delayed initiation of sexual intercourse contributed equally to declining adolescent pregnancy rates [11]. In the United States, there has been an increased use of condoms and an increased use of long-acting hormonal methods such as depot medroxyprogesterone acetate (DMPA) and the combination contraceptive patch, with a resultant decline in method-related contraceptive failures [10].

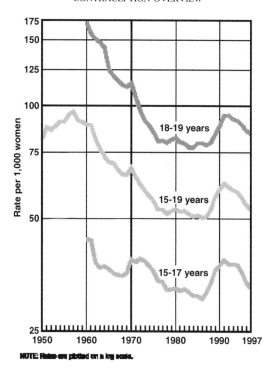

Fig. 2. Adolescent birth rate, 1950 to 1997. National Center for Vital Statistics Report, Vol. 47, No. 12, December 17, 1998.

Data from the most recently reported NSFG indicated that somewhat more than 20% of 15-year-olds have had intercourse and thus remain at risk for pregnancy [13]. The younger the adolescent is at the time of sexual initiation, the more likely she is to have more partners over her lifetime [13]. This statistic is complicated, however, by the fact that younger adolescents are more likely to

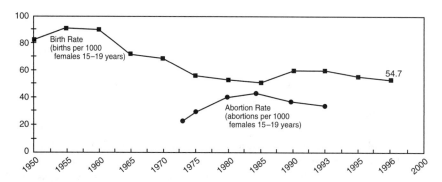

Fig. 3. Trends in birth rates and abortion rates among adolescent females aged 15 to 19 years. (*From* American Academy of Pediatrics Committee on Adolescence. Adolescent pregnancy—current trends and issues: 1998. Pediatrics 1999;103(2):516–803.)

have a partner who is significantly older than they and are more likely to have had unwanted or coerced sexual activity [13]. Among adolescents younger than 18, two thirds of those with a partner 6 or more years older used contraction at most recent sex, compared with 78% of those with a partner within 2 years of their own age [14]. For these reasons and because of many other psychosocial and developmental factors, the youngest teens are most likely to be ineffective users of contraception.

There has been less progress in improving US rates of adolescent pregnancy than among many other countries [15]. Other countries have addressed adolescent pregnancy with better access to health care and contraceptive services, better sexuality education, and higher rates of contraceptive use, especially oral contraceptives [16].

Although it is clear that adolescent pregnancy impacts the individual adolescent (and her partner, to a lesser degree), her infant, and society, unintended pregnancy is a problem for women of all ages. Adolescent pregnancies make up only about 21% of all unintended pregnancies in the United States [17]. Babies born to teen mothers are more likely to be premature and of low birth weight with the myriad of medical problems that entails, less likely to finish high school and more likely to do poorly in school, more likely to be abused or neglected. The sons are more likely to go to prison, and the daughters are more likely to themselves be teen mothers [18]. Two thirds of families begun by unwed adolescent mothers live in poverty; almost half of all teen mothers and more than three quarters of unmarried teen mothers receive welfare within 5 years of the birth. Teen childbearing costs taxpayers approximately $7 billion per year in direct costs for health care, foster care, criminal justice, public assistance, and lost tax revenues [18].

Adolescent medical care for contraception/confidentiality

Adolescents typically wait 1 year or more after initiating sexual intercourse before seeking medical advice about contraception [17]. More recent data from the early 1990s suggest that the median time from initiation of intercourse until the first family planning visit is 22 months, a percentage that had increased somewhat over time, largely because of increases in the reliance on provider-independent methods of contraception (primarily condoms) [19,23].

It has been estimated that 50% of adolescent pregnancies occur within the first 6 months after the initiation of sexual intercourse [20]. Adolescents are starting to get the messages about the need for contraception in spite of abstinence curricula that may not address contraception, leaving considerable knowledge gaps. In the early 1980s, more than half (52%) of adolescents used no method of contraception at the time of first intercourse [21]. This reflects the mixed messages about sexuality that adolescents receive in the United States: good girls do not have intercourse, and that to have unplanned intercourse is less morally reprehensible than to plan to have sex using effective contraception. In the 1980s, however, adolescents began to hear about the use of condoms, which were discussed primarily with regard to minimizing the risks of acquiring sexually transmitted diseases and HIV rather than preventing pregnancy. A discussion of condoms for contraception remained off-limits, but the use of condoms for sexually transmitted disease (STD) protection and contraception has increased over time. The 1988 method at the time of first intercourse, according to the National Survey of Family Growth was the first national survey to assess such dual use [22]. By the mid-1990s, only 23% of adolescents reported the use of no method at the time of first intercourse, according to the National Survey of Family Growth [23].

Adolescent contraceptive choices

Contraceptive choices of adolescents have changed over time, and there are numerous determinants of contraceptive use among adolescents [24,25]. Age is an important determinant of contraceptive use, and younger teens are less likely to use contraception at first intercourse. Black and Hispanic females are as likely to use contraception as white females. Socioeconomic status also is associated with contraceptive use; teens of higher socioeconomic status (as evidenced by their mother's educational attainment) are more likely to delay the initiation of intercourse and to use effective contraception. Parental education and family structure (eg, growing up in a two-parent household) influence the initiation of intercourse and condom use. Religious affiliation and religiosity influence the initiation of intercourse; teens who describe themselves as strongly religious are less likely to have early sex but are also less likely to use contraception at first intercourse.

Data for adolescent use of contraception are available from the 1995 cycle of the NSFG [24,25]. Approximately 97% of all teens have used some method of contraception and are trying to prevent pregnancies. Ninety-four percent have used condoms. Oral contraceptives have been used by 52% of teens surveyed. Forty-three percent of teens have used a relatively ineffective method—withdrawal—to prevent pregnancy. Thirteen percent of teens have relied on periodic abstinence for birth control, although studies suggest that many adolescents cannot identify the most fertile time of their cycle. Adolescents are using dual methods, that is, relying on hormonal contraceptives to minimize the risk of pregnancy and barrier methods to minimize the risks of acquiring STDs. The 1988 NSFG was the first national survey to incorporate questions about dual method use [26]. One report found that the highest rates of dual use of condoms plus another method occurred among oral contraceptive users [27]. Dual use among adolescents has increased over time as evidenced in the Youth Risk Behavior Survey (YRBS), with older students more likely to use condoms and another method; however, dual use remains low, at 7% [28].

Oral contraceptive use as assessed in the NSFG declined from 43% in 1988 to 25% of sexually active teens in 1995; condom use rose from 31% to 38%; long-acting/injectable methods rose to 7% [25]. Unfortunately, the use of no method rose from 20% to 29% [25].

Patterns of contraceptive use also contribute to contraceptive efficacy. More than two-thirds of adolescents aged 15 to 19 years reported long-term uninterrupted contraceptive use; however, they are more likely than older women to report sporadic use and less likely to report uninterrupted use of a very effective method of contraception (implant, injectable, intrauterine device [IUD], or oral contraceptives) [29]. Contraceptive use pattern was found to more strongly correlate with unintended pregnancy than did contraceptive use at first intercourse. Among adolescents initiating intercourse between the ages of 15 and 19, half of those who did not use a contraceptive became pregnant compared with 13% of those who did; 85% of long-term nonusers became pregnant within 12 months compared with 33% of sporadic users and fewer than 15% of uninterrupted users [29].

Newer methods of contraception

Newer methods have become available that take advantage of technologies that do not require daily pill taking. It has been estimated that incorrect or inconsistent use or discontinuation of oral contraceptives results in approximately 1 million unintended pregnancies per year in the United States [30]. Contraceptive options developed in the last 10 years include: the transdermal patch, the progestin-containing intrauterine system, the combination estrogen–progestin vaginal ring, and the combination estrogen–progestin intramuscular monthly injection. The last option has been taken off the market because of manufacturing-related concerns. One other long-acting method that was popular among adolescents and whose use is reflected in the NSFG and YRBS was levonorgestrel subdermal implant, which is also no longer available. Liability issues led to its withdrawal, in spite of data showing ongoing effectiveness, satisfaction, popularity, and use among adolescents. A single rod implant has undergone extensive testing with a demonstrated Pearl index of 0 pregnancies per 100 woman years. It has been available in Europe since 1999 and was issued an approvable letter by the US Food and Drug Administration (FDA) in November 2004; thus it likely will be available in the near future.

Long-acting hormonal contraceptive methods with low failure rates— the implant and the injectable—became available in the 1990s, accounting for 13% of current contraceptive users by 1995. The declining rates of adolescent pregnancy during the 1990s have been attributed in large part to the shift to long-acting methods, with a resultant increase in overall contraceptive effectiveness [10]. Although the contraceptive implant is no longer available, it is hoped that the increasing use of the other less compliance-dependent methods—the patch, the vaginal ring, and the injectable—will allow for a continuation of the trends in adolescent pregnancy rates.

In years past, one suggested goal of contraceptive development has been that the method would have little or no effect on the menstrual cycle. More specifically, it has been felt to be desirable to mimic a normal 28-day cycle. Combination oral contraceptives have thus been formulated in a manner to provide an artificial but typically regular monthly cycle. Effects such as breakthrough bleeding contribute to method dissatisfaction and discontinuation [31]. For many years, however, clinicians have used hormonal manipulation of the menstrual cycle to provide therapeutic amenorrhea for individuals with underlying medical problems [32]. Oral contraceptives, depot medroxyprogesterone acetate, and more recently levonorgestrel-containing intrauterine systems have been used in this fashion. In addition, a new packaging of an old combination oral contraceptive formulation has been marketed as containing 84 days of hormonally active pills followed by 7 placebo pills, leading to four periods a year. The desirability of an extended cycle hormonal method is not universal; however, some adolescents may prefer to have fewer menstrual cycles, minimizing menstrual-related symptoms and premenstrual molimina. The impact of this newer option on contraceptive use and compliance among adolescents is not established. Breakthrough bleeding is common in the first few months of use, which may lead to pill discontinuation.

Emergency contraception (EC) can be used when a method fails (such as a condom that breaks or slips off) or when no method of contraception is used. If EC is used in these situations, it has been estimated that approximately 1 million abortions and 2 million pregnancies ending in childbirth could be prevented per year in the United States [33]. Increased access to EC with over-the-counter (OTC) sales was supported by over 70 medical organizations including the American Academy of Pediatrics (AAP), American College of Obstetricians and Gynecologists (ACOG), American Medical Association (AMA), and American Academy of Family Physicians (AAFP). Two FDA advisory panels supported OTC availability. Unfortunately, the panels' recommendations and medical science were overlooked in favor of what most scientists consider to be political decision-making, and the company's application to the FDA for OTC status was denied [34]. In response to the FDA's actions, the company's proposed restrictions on the availability based on age may be successful in allowing the availability of EC for those over the age of 16.

Effects of contraception on sexual behavior and risks

Although FDA officials expressed concerns about the unknown potential health risks of ECs for young adolescents and concern about the effects of ECs on sexual behaviors, studies have shown that adolescents are not more likely to engage in risky behaviors such as unprotected intercourse, or less condom or hormonal contraceptive use if they have an advance prescription for ECs available for use [35]. Instead, they were more likely to use EC when needed, and to use it sooner, when it will be more effective than if they needed to contact a health care provider for a prescription.

The use of both a hormonal method of contraception to minimize the risks of pregnancy and condoms to minimize the risks of STDs—dual method use approach—has been investigated. Oral contraceptive users are more likely to use a dual method approach than are users of other contraceptive methods [28]. The type of partner (causal or main) and perceived STD risk influence dual use [36]. Adolescents are less likely to use condoms in addition to hormonal contraception with their main partner than with casual partners because of perceived lower risk of STDs. An awareness of the impact of relationship differences on contraceptive and risk-taking behaviors will enable clinicians to better counsel and advise adolescents.

References

[1] Darroch JE, Frost J, Singh S, et al. Teenage sexual and reproductive behavior in developed countries: can more progress be made? New York: The Alan Guttmacher Institute; 2001.

[2] National Campaign to Prevent Teen Pregnancy. Fact sheet: how is the thirty-four percent calculated? National Campaign to Prevent Teen Pregnancy. Available at: http://www.teenpregnancy.org/resources/reading/pdf/35percent.pdf. Accessed November 29, 2004.

[3] Henshaw SK. US teenage pregnancy statistics with comparative statistics for women aged 20–24. New York: The Alan Guttmacher Institute; 2004.

[4] Hamilton B, Martin JA, Sutton P. Births: preliminary data for 2003. Hyattsville (MD): National Center for Health Statistics; 2004.

[5] Henshaw SK. Unintended pregnancy in the United States. Fam Plann Perspect 1998;30(1):24–9.

[6] Stevens-Simon C, Beach RK, Klerman LV. To be rather than not to be—that is the problem with the questions we ask adolescents about their childbearing intentions. Arch Pediatr Adolesc Med Dec 2001;155(12):1298–300.

[7] Moore KA, Miller BC, Sugland BW, et al. Beginning too soon: adolescent sexual behavior, pregnancy, and parenthood. Washington (DC): Child Trends; 1995.

[8] Bachrach CA, Stolley KS, London KA. Relinquishment of premarital births: evidence from national survey data. Fam Plann Perspect 1992;24:27–32, 48.

[9] Darroch JE. Adolescent pregnancy trends and demographics. Curr Womens Health Rep 2001; 1(2):102–10.

[10] Darroch JE, Singh S. Why is teenage pregnancy declining? The roles of abstinence, sexual activity, and contraceptive use. New York: The Alan Guttmacher Institute; 1999.

[11] Santelli JS, Abma J, Ventura S, et al. Can changes in sexual behaviors among high school students explain the decline in teen pregnancy rates in the 1990s? J Adolesc Health 2004; 35(2):80–90.

[12] Strauss LT, Herndon J, Chang J, et al. Abortion Surveillance—United Sates, 2001. Atlanta (GA): Centers for Disease Control and Prevention; November 26, 2004;53(SS09):1–32.

[13] Abma JC, Chandra A, Mosher WD, et al. Fertility, family planning, and women's health: new data from the 1995 National Survey of Family Growth. Vital Health Stat 1997;23(19):1–114.

[14] Darroch JE, Landry DJ, Oslak S. Age differences between sexual partners in the United States. Fam Plann Perspect 1999;31(4):160–7.

[15] UNICEF. A league table of teenage births in rich nations. Florence (Italy): Innocenti Research Center; 2001.

[16] Darroch JE, Singh S, Frost JJ. Differences in teenage pregnancy rates among five developed countries: the roles of sexual activity and contraceptive use. Fam Plann Perspect 2001;33(6): 244–50.

[17] The Alan Guttmacher Institute. Sex and America's teenagers. New York: The Alan Guttmacher Institute; 1994.

[18] The National Campaign to Prevent Teen Pregnancy. Teen pregnancy. General facts and stats. Available at: http://www.teenpregnancy.org/resources/data/genlfact.asp. Accessed December 2, 2004.

[19] Finer LB, Zabin LS. Does the timing of the first family planning visit still matter? Fam Plann Perspect 1998;30(1):30–3.

[20] Zabin LS, Kantner JF, Zelnik M. The risk of adolescent pregnancy in the first months of intercourse. Fam Plann Perspect 1979;11(4):215–22.

[21] Mosher WD, McNally JW. Contraceptive use at first premarital intercourse: United States, 1965–1988. Fam Plann Perspect 1991;23(3):108–16.

[22] Piccinino LJ, Mosher WD. Trends in contraceptive use in the United States: 1982–1995. Fam Plann Perspect 1998;30(1):4–10.

[23] Manning WD, Longmore MA, Giordano PC. The relationship context of contraceptive use at first intercourse. Fam Plann Perspect 2000;32(3):104–10.

[24] Piccinino LJ, Mosher WD. Trends in contraceptive use in the United States: 1982–1995. Fam Plann Perspect 1998;30:4–10.

[25] Abma JC, Sonenstein FL. Sexual activity and contraceptive practices among teenagers in the United States, 1988 and 1995. Vital Health Stat 2001;23(21):1–87.

[26] Bankole A, Darroch JE, Singh S. Determinants of trends in condom use in the United States, 1988–1995. Fam Plann Perspect 1999;31(6):264–71.

[27] Santelli JS, Warren CW, Lowry R, et al. The use of condoms with other contraceptive methods among young men and women. Fam Plann Perspect 1997;29(6):261–7.

[28] Anderson JE, Santelli J, Gilbert BC. Adolescent dual use of condoms and hormonal contraception: trends and correlates 1991–2001. Sex Transm Dis 2003;30(9):719–22.

[29] Glei DA. Measuring contraceptive use patterns among teenage and adult women. Fam Plann Perspect 1999;31(2):73–80.

[30] Rosenberg MJ, Waugh MS, Long S. Unintended pregnancies and use, misuse and discontinuation of oral contraceptives. J Reprod Med 1995;40:355–60.

[31] Hillard PJ. The patient's reaction to side effects of oral contraceptives. Am J Obstet Gynecol 1989;161:1412–5.

[32] Hillard PJ. Therapeutic amenorrhea. J Pediatr Hematol Oncol 1999;21(5):350–3.

[33] Trussell J, Stewart F. The effectiveness of postcoital hormonal contraception. Fam Plann Perspect 1992;24:262–4.

[34] Grimes DA. Emergency contraception: politics trumps science at the US Food and Drug Administration. Obstet Gynecol 2004;104(2):220–1.

[35] Gold MA, Wolford JE, Smith KA, et al. The effects of advance provision of emergency contraception on adolescent women's sexual and contraceptive behaviors. J Pediatr Adolesc Gynecol 2004;17(2):87–96.

[36] Ott MA, Adler NE, Millstein SG, et al. The trade-off between hormonal contraceptives and condoms among adolescents. Perspect Sex Reprod Health 2002;34(1):6–14.

ELSEVIER
SAUNDERS

ADOLESCENT
MEDICINE
CLINICS

Adolesc Med 16 (2005) 495–515

Barrier and Spermicidal Contraceptives in Adolescence

Jenna McNaught, MD, FRCSC, Mary Anne Jamieson, MD, FRCSC*

Department of Obstetrics and Gynecology, Queen's University, Victory 4, Kingston General Hospital, 76 Stuart Street, Kingston, Ontario K7L 2V7, Canada

Barriers are a class of contraception that prevents pregnancy by providing a physical or chemical barrier to keep sperm from entering the cervix. This is the oldest form of contraception; ancient writings refer to intravaginal sponges, leaves, seaweed, and pastes. Egyptian papyri from 1850 BC refer to mixtures of honey, acacia, and crocodile dung that were placed in the vagina before intercourse [1]. The ancient Egyptians also wore decorative sheaths over their penises as early as 1350 BC [2]. Penile sheaths made of linen were described in 1564 AD by Italian anatomist Fallopius [2] and were designed initially to "protect the penis" from infection rather than prevent pregnancy [1]. In the 1700s, condoms made from animal intestines were used for contraception as well [1]. With the invention of vulcanized rubber in the 1840s, synthetic rubber condoms were produced [2]. Other vaginal barrier methods subsequently followed in the late 19th century [1].

Because they prevent semen from contacting the cervix, upper genital tract, and, depending on the method, the vaginal mucosa, barrier methods generally offer some degree of protection against sexually transmitted infections (STIs) in addition to their contraceptive properties. They are nonhormonal, with essentially no systemic effects, but because barriers are coitally dependent, they can have substantial failure rates with typical use. These methods are more susceptible to user error because they depend on proper placement and consistent

* Corresponding author.
E-mail address: maj3@post.queensu.ca (M.A. Jamieson).

1547-3368/05/$ – see front matter © 2005 Elsevier Inc. All rights reserved.
doi:10.1016/j.admecli.2005.06.002
adolescent.theclinics.com

use to be effective. As a result, there can be a large difference between "typical" and "perfect use" failure rates.

Failure rates in trials of barrier contraceptives generally are reported as 6- or 12-month cumulative life-table probabilities of pregnancy. Although expressed as a percentage, this is not the same as the Pearl index, defined as the number of pregnancies per 100 women-years. Furthermore, because proper use of a barrier method depends on user skill, the failure rates are highest in the first months of use and improve as the person gains experience, or as unmotivated users drop out of the cohort by stopping the method or conceiving. Therefore, one cannot merely double a 6-month failure rate to get the 12-month rate (which would allow comparisons with other contraceptive methods more easily). Unfortunately, many research trials involving barrier methods are conducted over 6 months and the 12-month failure rates reported often are calculated from the 6-month data. Thus the data on the efficacy of barrier methods are less than ideal for comparisons, and there can be a wide range of failure rates depending on the underlying fertility of the population studied, among other factors.

Because of their dependence on a motivated and skilled user having somewhat planned intercourse, barrier methods may not be used as successfully by teenaged patients nor viewed as positively by them. Nonetheless, teenagers should be encouraged to use condoms for STI protection, even if they are using another contraceptive method (so-called "dual protection").

The male condom

The male condom (Fig. 1) is one of the most well-known and widely used forms of contraception [3]. It is a thin, tight-fitting sheath that is unrolled to the base of the penis, covering the shaft completely. The semen is trapped inside and is prevented from contacting any part of the female genital tract. In addition to preventing pregnancy therefore, the condom also prevents STIs that are carried in semen such as gonorrhea, chlamydia, trichomonas, HIV, and hepatitis B. With regard to the human papilloma virus (HPV), condoms seem to offer some protection against genital warts and cervical dysplasia/cancer but not against HPV infection overall, likely because much of the genital area is not covered [4]. A 2002 Cochrane review [5] showed that consistent condom use reduced HIV transmission among serodiscordant heterosexual couples by 80%. The latex condom's role in reducing STIs and HIV transmission is well established [6], and thus it has a unique and valuable role in family planning and public health efforts, even if couples also are using another method of contraception. Condoms can be used by any couple wanting to prevent pregnancy or STI.

There is a wide variety of condoms on the market today, with various shapes, textures, colors, and flavors. They vary in thickness from 0.03 to 0.1 mm [2,7], and there are latex (most common) and nonlatex varieties such as poly-

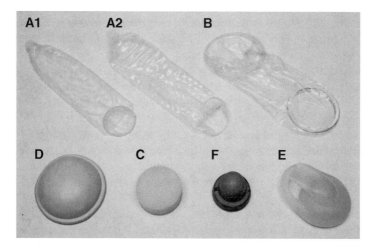

Fig. 1. Barrier methods. (*A*) Male condoms: (*A1*) latex, (*A2*) polyurethane. (*B*) Female condom. (*C*) Contraceptive sponge. (*D*) Diaphragm. (*E*) Lea's Shield. (*F*) Cervical cap. (Photo by C. Peck, Medical Photography Services, Queen's University, Kingston, ON, Canada.)

urethane, synthetic elastomers, and lambskin. Lambskin is permeable to viral particles and should be used only for contraception, not for prevention of infection [6].

Efficacy

Pregnancy rates are quoted as 2% per year for perfect use and 15% per year for typical use [8]. Condoms are therefore the most effective of the barrier methods. Condoms can break or slip, but it is believed that most failures are a result of improper or inconsistent use (user error) rather than condom failure [6,9,10]. Breakage can result from improper handling or storage, use of oil-based lubricants, use past the expiration date, not leaving a reservoir at the tip, or from vaginal dryness [2,10]. Slippage has been associated with excessive lubricant use in some studies and with improper handling during withdrawal [11]. This also may be a problem with nonlatex condoms (see later discussion).

One prospective study of heterosexual couples that were not relying on condoms for pregnancy or STI protection reported that 7.9% of condoms either broke or slipped off during intercourse [11]. The same investigators, in another trial with the same design, found that only 1.46% of condoms either broke or fell off. They attributed the much lower rate to more precise wording in the second study [12]. Condoms also can slip off during withdrawal, but this is considered user error and was not included in the above numbers. Another trial reported a similar rate of 6.1% for breakage or slippage [13]. Retrospective studies report lower breakage rates. It is estimated that one pregnancy occurs for every 19 condom breaks [10]; therefore, emergency contraception should be offered.

Condoms lubricated with spermicide are available, but there is no evidence that they improve the contraceptive efficacy of the condom because the quantity of spermicide is low [14]. With this in mind, given the concerns regarding vaginal irritation and HIV transmission with frequent use of nonoxynol-9 (see later discussion), spermicidally lubricated condoms no longer are recommended, but they are obviously preferable to not using a condom at all [14]. Couples at low risk for HIV transmission who want to increase the condom's contraceptive effectiveness would be served better by using a separately applied vaginal spermicide, which in combination with condoms is believed to provide similar protection to the combined oral contraceptive pill [15]. Using a separate spermicide guarantees its presence in the vagina in the event of condom breakage [2].

It is important to educate users that only water-based lubricants are appropriate to use with latex condoms because oil-based lubricants degrade latex in as little as 60 seconds [16]. A common misperception is that hand lotions are water-based because they wash off with water, but they contain mineral oil and thus should not be used with latex. Many vaginal medications are also oil-based [2].

Recently, the development of nonlatex condoms has provided a contraceptive option to couples where one of the partners is allergic to latex. Polyurethane is a durable plastic that is impermeable to sexually transmitted pathogens including HIV [17,18]. Oil-based lubricants can be used with nonlatex condoms. In vitro, polyurethane seems to be stronger than latex and less prone to degradation, but in clinical use, polyurethane condoms (marketed under brand names Avanti, Trojan Supra, and eZ.on) have higher rates of slippage and breakage [19,20]. There may be a slight difference in pregnancy rates between brands of polyurethane condoms [20–22].

A trial of 805 monogamous couples randomized to using either a latex or polyurethane condom exclusively for 6 months showed that clinical failure (defined as breaking or slipping off completely during intercourse or withdrawal) was higher in the polyurethane group for the first five uses of the condom (8.5% versus 1.6%; relative risk [RR] 5.2) and after 6 months (3.6% versus 0.9%; RR 4.3) [19]. The observed 6-month pregnancy rates were not significantly different, but this could have been related to the higher discontinuation rate in the polyurethane group. The men preferred the latex condoms overall, although they were more likely to report penile compression with the latex condom, and they preferred the polyurethane condom's lack of odor. Some users perceived improved sensitivity with the polyurethane condom, but the trend was not statistically significant.

Another new nonlatex alternative is the Tactylon condom, made from a synthetic elastomer used to make nonlatex gloves. This material is reported to be hypoallergenic and to have similar elastic properties to latex, but has a longer shelf life [23]. In one trial, the combined breakage and slippage rates between a Tactylon and a latex condom were not different (1.9%) [12]. In a larger trial, however, three different styles of Tactylon condom each had significantly higher breakage rates (3.75% average) than the standard latex condom (0.86%) but equivalent slippage rates. Men and women preferred the two US Food and Drug Administration (FDA)–approved styles of Tactylon condoms (Standard and Low-Modulus) to the latex condom, and there were fewer medical events (irritation, burning, itching, or genital pain) with these nonlatex condoms [23].

Clinical failure rates (breakage or slippage) are used as surrogate markers for efficacy in most trials because increased exposure to bodily fluids could increase pregnancy rates and STI transmission. A reduction in STI transmission in clinical use has not been well studied for nonlatex condoms. Given the increased rates of clinical failure with nonlatex condoms, it would seem prudent to recommend latex condoms as the criterion standard. Even so, common sense suggests that polyurethane and Tactylon condoms still can protect against pregnancy and infection and should be recommended for the latex-allergic couple, or based on personal preference (as opposed to using no condom at all). These condoms are often more expensive than latex condoms.

Advantages

Condoms are relatively inexpensive, safe, accessible, and easy to use. They may help prolong intercourse. Condoms are the only reversible form of contraception (aside from withdrawal) that involves the male partner in making healthy sexual choices. Like all barrier methods, there are no systemic effects, and they only are used when coitally active. Latex condoms reduce STI transmission in addition to their contraceptive efficacy.

Disadvantages

Disadvantages include interruption of intimacy and possible decreased sensation for some male partners. Dependence on the male partner, and on an erection, also can be drawbacks. Some men find it difficult to maintain an erection with a condom on. Either partner may experience genital irritation. A reaction to condoms is not always caused by a latex allergy; it also can be a result of the spermicide or the lubricant. Men and women who are allergic to latex can use nonlatex condoms as discussed previously.

Tips for proper use and patient counseling

It sometimes is assumed that all men know how to use a condom, but this is not true. Men and women should be instructed properly. Proper use entails putting on the condom soon after the penis is erect, before any genital contact. The condom should be removed carefully from the package, avoiding tearing from nails, rings, and other contact. The condom then is set on the tip of the penis with the rolled side up. The tip should be pinched to expel air and leave a reservoir to collect the semen. The other hand rolls the condom down to the base of the penis. After ejaculation, the penis must be withdrawn right away, holding the base of the condom to avoid slipping. Away from his partner's body, the man should remove the condom and throw it away. A new condom should be used for each act of intercourse. It is important to be explicit to avoid misuse. For instance, some people unroll the condom and fill it with water to check for leakage, and then slide it on the penis like a sock.

Troubleshooting

1. Decreased sensation: try putting a drop of lubricant or saliva on the inside of the condom to increase friction. Textured or ultra-thin condoms may also help.
2. Spoiling the mood: make putting on the condom a part of foreplay.
3. Condom breakage: immediately insert vaginal spermicide if available, and consider emergency contraception. Always keep an extra condom on hand in case of breakage.
4. Latex allergy: try a nonlubricated, nonspermicidal condom first because latex may not be causing the reaction. Otherwise, use a nonlatex condom. Remember that lambskin condoms can be used for pregnancy prevention but do not prevent STIs.
5. Trouble convincing partner to use a condom: rehearse the scenarios in Table 1, and visit www.plannedparenthood.org for more information.

When used properly, the latex male condom offers pregnancy prevention and superior STI protection. This makes condoms an ideal choice for teenagers, especially when combined with a more reliable form of contraception. Motivation and ready access are essential for their use, however, and unfortunately lack of these is often a limiting factor. The new nonlatex condoms offer these benefits to latex-allergic couples, or those who find latex condoms distasteful,

Table 1
Scenarios for condom negotiation

When your partner says...	You can say...
"I don't have any infections."	"That's good, neither do I as far as I know. But either of us could have an infection and not know it so it's safer if we use a condom."
"If you loved me, you wouldn't ask me to wear one."	"It's because I love you that I want us both to be protected."
"I can't feel anything with a condom on."	"Let's try putting some lubrication in the condom. I've read that can help."
	"If you don't wear a condom you won't feel anything!"
"I'm too embarrassed to buy them."	"Let's go together. We can make a game of it. It'll be fun!"
"I can't believe you brought a condom! Were you expecting that we'd have sex?"	"I always carry a condom with me because I like to be prepared. It doesn't mean we have to have sex, or that I expected it."
"I don't have one with me."	"I do."

but for the average couple, and on a population level, latex condoms should be recommended.

The female condom

The female condom (see Fig. 1) is a pliable polyurethane sheath that has a smaller, unattached, flexible inner ring in the closed end and a larger outer ring at the open end. The inner ring is inserted high into the vagina and helps hold it in place. The outer ring remains on the vulva so that the condom forms a sheath completely lining the vagina. The penis is inserted into the sheath during coitus, so there is a barrier between the penis and the vagina, cervix, and part of the vulva. The inside of the condom is prelubricated with a silicone-based lubricant.

The female condom is marketed in North America under the brand name FC Female Condom (formerly Reality). Like male condoms, it is available in drug stores without a prescription and each condom is intended for a single use. It costs slightly more than the male condom: approximately $ 2.50 per condom [24].

Efficacy

The female condom has a first-year failure rate of 5% with perfect use and 21% with typical use [8] and thus is comparable to the diaphragm but not as reliable as the male condom. These rates are based on the largest efficacy trial involving 328 American and Latin American women that reported 6-month probabilities of pregnancy of 12.4% and 22.2%, respectively, for typical use (approximately 15% overall), and 2.6% and 9.5%, respectively, for perfect use [25]. The women from Latin America were more likely to be parous, younger, and less educated. Because they also had less prior experience with barrier methods, no population-based comparisons could be drawn. The 12-month failure rates were calculated from the 6-month data based on known differences between the first and second 6 months of use of other barrier methods [26].

Smaller trials have demonstrated somewhat better efficacy. One of the first trials, conducted in the United Kingdom, reported a 15% probability of pregnancy in 12 months of typical use [27]. A study of 190 Japanese women reported better success; the 6-month probability of pregnancy was 3.2% with typical and 0.8% with perfect use [28].

The female condom was impermeable to HIV and other sexually transmitted pathogens in laboratory testing [17,18]. It is believed to be similar to the male condom in providing protection from vaginal/cervical infections and HIV, but there is limited clinical evidence for this claim [29–31]. Establishing reduced STI rates with the female condom has been problematic because the male condom is so effective at reducing HIV transmission that it is considered unethical to randomize people at risk for acquiring HIV to any option that excludes male condoms. One study showed that there were fewer leaks and less slippage/dislodgement with the female condom (3% versus 11.6% with the male condom), which resulted in less vaginal exposure to semen [13]. In another study, women at an STI clinic were randomized by the week of their visit to education about either the male or female condom and were given free supplies of that condom for up to 12 months [29]. The investigators looked at incidence rates of syphilis, gonorrhea, chlamydia, and trichomonas for the women who came back to the clinic. The authors found a reduction in STIs favoring the group given female condoms, but the findings were not statistically significant (odds ratio 0.75; 95% confidence interval [CI] 0.56–1.01), and the methodology had some scientific limitations.

Because the female condom covers some of the vulva, it may reduce transmission of pathogens such as the herpes simplex virus, HPV, and syphilis, which are spread through skin-to-skin contact [32].

Advantages

Because this method is controlled by the woman and is less constricting to the penis, it may be helpful in situations where a man refuses to wear a condom. Unlike the male condom, it does not depend on the man having an erection. It can be inserted as long as 8 hours before coitus, which can improve spontaneity [33]. The female condom can be obtained without a prescription or physician visit. Breakage rates are lower than those of the male condom [13,34], and the nonlatex female condom can be used with oil-based lubricants, whereas latex barriers cannot.

Disadvantages

The cost may be prohibitive for some potential users, and the product can sometimes make a distracting noise during coitus. Slippage of the condom is one problem that may account for some failures, especially for new users [34]. Difficulties with insertion and discomfort from the inner ring also have been reported [35]. The woman must be able to insert the inner ring high up in the vagina.

Acceptability and STI transmission rates of the female condom have been studied extensively in developing countries, especially with sex-trade workers. In one report of Thai sex workers, the number of sex acts where a condom was worn was similarly high between the control group encouraged to use male condoms as usual and the experimental group supplied with female condoms as a back-up option (97%–98% in each group). In the experimental group, the use of male condoms decreased proportionately to an increase in female condom use. The authors concluded that these women were less insistent on male condoms because they had a back-up method available, and the increased use of the female condom suggested that it could be more appealing to the workers or their clients in some situations. The female condom had less breakage, which reduced the overall number of unprotected sex acts. There was a nonsignificant decrease in STIs in the female + male condom group [34].

Acceptability has varied depending on the population studied but has been fairly positive overall, ranging from 41% to 95% [35,36]. Some women, particularly teenagers, may not like it because of its blatancy during sex and issues related to comfort with insertion. Failure rates have reportedly been higher in women younger than 25 years of age [26]. The female condom may benefit some women, however, and may help in situations where a woman otherwise might have no other option for protection. One of the most important features of the female condom is the empowerment it offers women. International family planning agencies are looking at the feasibility of reusing female condoms to reduce costs, especially for developing countries [36].

Tips for proper use and patient counseling

The woman inserts the inner ring into the vagina before intercourse. When penetration occurs, care must be taken to ensure that the penis enters the sheath. After ejaculation, the man does not need to withdraw right away as with a male condom. The female condom is removed by twisting the outer ring to trap the semen inside and then pulling it out before standing up. It should not be used simultaneously with a male condom because the resultant friction may increase slippage or breakage [37].

Spermicides

Spermicides consist of a spermicidal agent in a vehicle that allows its distribution throughout the vagina. Almost all available spermicides contain

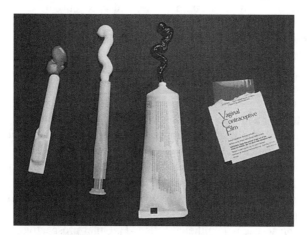

Fig. 2. Spermicides (from left to right): spermicidal cream, foam, gel, and film. (Photo by C. Peck, Medical Photography Services, Queen's University, Kingston, ON, Canada.)

nonoxynol-9 as their active spermicidal ingredient. These detergent-like compounds kill sperm by disrupting the cell membrane, causing water influx and lysis. There are several delivery systems available such as creams, gels, foams, vaginal suppositories, and a dissolvable vaginal film (Fig. 2). The vaginal film is a 5-cm × 5-cm piece of plastic that looks like waxed paper. Typical doses of nonoxynol 9 range from 50 to 150 mg per use [14].

Efficacy

Although spermicides are a heterogeneous group of products, it is unknown whether contraceptive properties differ between them. When used on their own as contraceptives, spermicides have a failure rate of approximately 29% for the first year with typical use and 18% with perfect use [8], although the reported range is large [38]. One multinational randomized trial comparing 72 mg of nonoxynol-9 in a vaginal film with 100 mg of nonoxynol-9 in a foaming tablet extrapolated their findings to predict a 12-month failure rate of 40% versus 44%, respectively, with no significant difference between the groups. In both groups, these high failure rates might be attributed to the study population, who were largely under 25 years of age with more than 10 acts of coitus per month [39].

Although spermicides may be less effective on their own, they can be valuable when used in combination with another barrier method. Kestelman [15] proved using a mathematical model that the contraceptive efficacy of using a male condom correctly along with a separately applied vaginal spermicide is comparable to that of the combined oral contraceptive, although this has not been proven in head-to-head studies.

Advantages

Spermicides are easy to obtain and use, and need only be used with coitus. They are nonhormonal, can be combined with any other method, and they are under the woman's control, without necessarily involving her partner. They also can provide some lubrication.

Disadvantages

Disadvantages include messiness (with the creams, gels, and foams), unpleasant taste/odor, the need to reapply with every act of intercourse, and the potential for vaginal irritation (see later discussion). Spermicides (particularly when combined with a diaphragm) have been associated with an increase in urinary tract infections [40] as a result of alterations in normal vaginal flora. In one experiment, nonoxynol-9 had much more antibacterial effect against lactobacilli than uropathogenic bacteria, and also enhanced the adherence of Escherichia coli to vaginal epithelial cells [41]. Other prospective cohort studies have demonstrated an increase in E coli bacteriuria as well as increased vaginal colonization with E coli and other gram-negative uropathogens [42,43].

Spermicides are user-dependent. Timing of application and coitus can be an issue. The woman should feel comfortable inserting the product and must be able to place it in the proper position. The film, suppositories, or bioadhesive gel may be preferred if messiness or vaginal discharge is a concern. The bioadhesive gel may be less disruptive to intimacy (see later discussion).

Precautions

Sensitivity to nonoxynol-9 in either partner is a contraindication, as is the uncommon vaginal anomaly that could interfere with placement.

In recent years, the effect of spermicides on HIV transmission has come under scrutiny. Nonoxynol-9 has microbicidal properties in vitro, and therefore it was hoped that it could offer protection against HIV and other STIs [14,44–46]. Studies have shown that not only is nonoxynol-9 not effective in preventing HIV transmission [44], but that it may enhance transmission. In one study of 892 HIV-negative female sex workers from developing countries who were randomized to using condoms with either a placebo gel or a gel containing 52.5 mg of nonoxynol-9, Van Damme and colleagues [45] showed a trend of increased HIV seroconversion among women using the spermicide (hazard ratio 1.5; 95% CI 1.0–2.2; $P = .047$). When they looked at frequency of use, the women who were using the spermicidal gel more than 3.5 times per day had a higher risk of contracting HIV (hazard ratio 1.8; 95% CI 1.0–3.2; $P = .03$) compared with placebo, whereas among those who used less gel there was no difference.

Another placebo-controlled trial of the nonoxynol-9 sponge versus a placebo cream among prostitutes in Nairobi reported an increase in vaginal ulcers and HIV seroconversion among the sponge users, but the latter increase was not significant with an adjusted hazard ratio of 1.6 and a 95% confidence interval that overlapped 1 (0.8–2.8). This was despite having the same number of sexual partners and the same proportion of partners who used condoms. The study was terminated early because these results were inconsistent with the hypothesis that nonoxynol-9 might decrease HIV transmission [46].

With regards to chlamydia, gonorrhea, and other STIs, the evidence is conflicting. In Cochrane meta-analyses [47,48], the overall risk for HIV or vaginal infections (including bacterial vaginosis and yeast) for women using nonoxynol-9 was not statistically different from placebo, but this spermicide significantly increased the risk for vaginal ulceration and lesions, which could enhance HIV transmission if exposed.

Because the studies showing an increase in HIV transmission were done on women at high risk for HIV acquisition and who used a large volume of spermicide, caution must be used in applying these results to the average woman using nonoxynol-9 for its intended use as a contraceptive. In 2002, the World Health Organization (WHO) released a statement about nonoxynol-9 that concluded that it should not be used to prevent HIV or STI transmission; in such cases a condom should be used. They suggested that women at high risk for HIV infection or women who have multiple daily acts of intercourse should not use nonoxynol-9 because of the potential for enhanced transmission. For the woman at low risk for HIV infection, however, spermicides can and should remain a contraceptive option. The WHO went on to advise that condoms lubricated with nonoxynol-9 no longer should be promoted, given these concerns and the lack of evidence that condoms lubricated with spermicide offer superior contraceptive efficacy over a nonspermicidal condom. Of course, a condom lubricated with spermicide is better than no condom at all [14].

Tips for proper use and patient counseling

Spermicides can be purchased over the counter and usually are displayed with condoms and other reproductive health products. The gels, foams, and creams come with their own applicator and can be inserted immediately before intercourse, but the vaginal film or suppositories need to be inserted at least 15 minutes before intercourse to ensure they are dissolved and distributed throughout the vagina. Because these products are effective for 1 hour (with the exception of the bioadhesive gel), a second dose is needed if coitus occurs more than 1 hour after insertion. A subsequent act of intercourse requires another application. These products should be inserted high up in the vagina near the cervix. The woman must not douche for at least 6 hours after intercourse. Because the different products vary slightly, the instructions that come with a product should be read and followed.

One unique product is a bioadhesive gel (Advantage 24) containing 52.5 mg of nonoxynol-9 per application that binds to the vaginal epithelium to hold it in place longer and slowly release spermicide over 24 hours. Unlike other spermicides, it can be inserted up to 24 hours before anticipated coitus, although there is some evidence that it is more effective when applied closer to intercourse [49]. Additional episodes of intercourse require repeat applications.

The contraceptive sponge

The contraceptive sponge (see Fig. 1) is a close relative of the spermicide family. Contraceptive sponges provide a physical barrier by absorbing semen, but their main method of action comes from the spermicide with which they are saturated. Two brands of contraceptive sponge are available in Canada, but neither is available in the United States. Both are disposable, made of poly-urethane foam, come in one size only, and are inserted high in the vagina to cover the cervix.

The Today sponge is dimpled on one side to fit against the cervix and has a ribbon on the other side for removal. It contains a high dose of nonoxynol-9 (1000 mg) but only 125 mg is released from the sponge [50]. It needs to be moistened with water before insertion. The Today sponge remains effective for up to 24 hours and allows for multiple acts of intercourse during that time without having to add more spermicide. The sponge should be left in for 6 hours after the last intercourse.

The Today sponge was taken off the market in 1995 because of manufacturing issues, and the new manufacturer (Allendale Pharmaceuticals, New Jersey) is awaiting reapproval from the FDA. It returned to the Canadian market in 2003, and many American women are buying it through the Internet for approximately $4.50 per sponge [51].

The Protectaid sponge can be purchased through the Internet from Canada. It has a flat discoid shape and comes premoistened with spermicide. A removal handle is cut into the sponge. It is effective for 12 hours of unlimited intercourse.

Efficacy

The sponge is less reliable in parous women [52]. For nulliparous women the failure rate is 9% with perfect use and 16% with typical use. In parous women these rates are 20% and 32%, respectively [8]. It is not clear why this device fails more often in parous women, but presumably it is related to mechanical issues with the parous vagina and cervix. One cohort study of the Protectaid sponge had a failure rate of 23% over 1 year with no difference based on parity [53]. Compared with the diaphragm in randomized controlled trials, the sponge is less effective at preventing pregnancy and has a higher discontinuation rate [50]. The 12-month cumulative life table pregnancy rates per 100 women were 17.4 for the sponge versus 12.8 for the diaphragm in an American trial and 24.5 versus 10.9, respectively, in a British trial [50]. In a retrospective subgroup analysis of the larger United States trial, one of the investigators found that this difference only applied to parous women [52].

Precautions

Because the sponge is primarily a vehicle for spermicide, the previous discussion about vaginal irritation in high-volume users applies. This is not the method of choice for a woman at high risk for HIV acquisition, but for an average-risk woman it is an option for contraception. Based on case reports there may be a small risk of toxic shock syndrome; therefore, it probably should not be used during menses [54].

Teenagers may like this method because it does not require a fitting or a prescription, and should the FDA reapprove this method, it will be easy to obtain. The sponge is more discreet than condoms yet easier to use than a diaphragm or cervical cap. It can be placed long before intercourse and offers prolonged protection without the need for extra spermicide insertion. Because most teenagers are nulliparous it can be reasonably effective, but it requires proper and consistent use and does not offer the STI protection of a condom.

Diaphragms

A diaphragm (see Fig. 1) is a soft flexible dome usually made of latex rubber (see later discussion). When properly placed in the vagina, it sits between the posterior fornix and the pubic bone, covering the cervix. This method requires a prescription and a fitting by an experienced health care professional, and it must be refitted after childbirth or with weight fluctuations of more than 10 pounds.

Each of the three types of diaphragms available comes in sizes from 55 mm to 95 mm in diameter. The coil spring type is the most common and has a flat silhouette when compressed. It can be used by most women who have good pelvic support, but is easier for parous women to use because it can be difficult to get the posterior edge behind the cervix [55]. This style has an applicator to aid insertion, but manual insertion is better because it allows proper placement to be verified. The arcing spring diaphragm forms an arc that can make it easier for a nulliparous woman to maneuver behind her cervix [1]. The wide seal diaphragm has a broader rim that reportedly improves the seal against the vaginal mucosa. Because it is made of silicone, women who have a latex allergy can use it. This type is only available on the Internet from the manufacturer's website [56].

To fit the diaphragm, a bimanual examination is performed to assess the vaginal and pelvic anatomy. The middle finger is pressed against the posterior fornix. The thumb is used to mark where the pubic bone contacts the index finger. The distance between this point and the tip of the middle finger is used as an approximate diameter of ring to try first, but several sizes should be tried to determine which fits best. When properly fit, the diaphragm sits behind the pubic bone but not too tightly; there should be approximately 0.5 cm of space. The diaphragm should not come out with a valsalva maneuver and should feel comfortable to the patient [33]. A set of fitting rings can be obtained from the manufacturer (Ortho-McNeil Pharmaceutical Inc., Raritan, New Jersey).

Efficacy

Diaphragms have a failure rate of 6% with perfect use and 16% with typical use [8]. Unlike the sponge or cervical cap, the failure rates do not differ based on parity [26,50,52].

There is not good evidence to support the concomitant use of spermicides, although this is common practice. Some have reported good success with an unfitted 60-mm diaphragm worn continuously without spermicide [57]. These women remove their diaphragm each day for cleaning, then reinsert it. Those who support this method believe that, by eliminating the mess and inconvenience of spermicide and by always having the device in situ, compliance is improved. The only randomized clinical trial to date found no significant difference in pregnancy rates for diaphragm use with or without spermicide [58]. There was a trend to higher pregnancy rates without spermicide (cumulative pregnancy rate 28.6 versus 21.2, respectively, per 100 women in the first year of typical use), but because this study was underpowered, no firm conclusions could be drawn. At present there is poor evidence to support the use of spermicide, but according to a 2003 Cochrane review [59], there is "no evidence to change the commonly recommended practice of using the diaphragm with spermicide."

Advantages

A diaphragm may be a good option for a motivated woman who is comfortable with insertion (as with all female barrier methods) and who wants to avoid systemic effects. It is woman-controlled and it can be inserted before intercourse, thus improving spontaneity.

By covering the cervix, the diaphragm may offer some protection against cervical infections, pelvic inflammatory disease, and cervical dysplasia [6,55]. Because much of the vaginal mucosa is left uncovered, however, it may not protect against other STIs, including HIV. This is being studied in developing countries [60].

Disadvantages

The diaphragm requires a physician visit and a prescription. Because a woman must have adequate pelvic muscle tone to retain the device, it cannot be used in women who have significant pelvic organ prolapse. Because of the use of spermicides, there can be some messiness and concerns about vaginal irritation. There is a theoretical and presumably rare risk of toxic shock syndrome.

As discussed previously, the diaphragm has been associated with an increase in urinary tract infections [40–43] related to alterations in the vaginal flora or from pressure on the urethra. Recurrent UTIs may be a relative contraindication to its use.

Tips for proper use and patient counseling

The woman places the diaphragm in the vagina up to 6 hours before anticipated intercourse. Spermicidal jelly is recommended for use along with the diaphragm (in the dome and around the rim) although good evidence for this is lacking [58,59]. The diaphragm must remain in place for at least 6 hours after the last intercourse for a maximum of 24 hours total. If there is subsequent intercourse, another application of spermicide is recommended. Once removed, it is washed with mild soap and water, dried, and stored in its case. Powder is no longer recommended.

Because it requires some skill and comfort to use, and because of its higher overall failure rate compared with other methods, including the male condom, the diaphragm is not generally considered a first-line contraceptive method for adolescents. Some young women are motivated to use it, however, and can do so successfully after being well informed and instructed [61,62].

Lea's Shield

Lea's Shield (see Fig. 1) is similar to a diaphragm in that it is an intravaginal method that covers the cervix and is intended for use with spermicidal jelly. Lea's Shield comes in one size and does not need to be fitted, although it does require a prescription. It can be purchased at Planned Parenthood, from health care providers, or from the manufacturer using the Internet at http://www.leasshield.com (after sending in a prescription).

Lea's Shield is made of silicone as opposed to latex. Its design is unique, featuring a one-way valve that allows air to escape during insertion, causing suction between the device and the cervix. Mucus and blood can escape, so it can be used during menses. There is a loop that acts as a handle for easier removal. It must be worn for 8 hours after last intercourse, but it can be worn up to 48 hours in total and repeat spermicide applications are not required.

Efficacy

The adjusted 6-month life table pregnancy rate is reportedly 5.6 per 100 with spermicide and 9.3 per 100 without spermicide [63], although the difference was not statistically significant. These rates give a projected 12-month failure rate of 15% for typical use, which is comparable to other barrier methods [64].

Advantages and disadvantages

Lea's Shield can be left in place longer than the diaphragm, without the need for further spermicide application. It is a nonlatex device. Its advantages and disadvantages are otherwise similar to the diaphragm.

Cervical caps

Cervical caps are designed to fit snugly over the cervix to prevent semen from entering. As such, they are smaller than diaphragms. Like diaphragms, cervical caps need to be fitted by an experienced health professional and refitted after pregnancy. The two devices approved by the FDA are the latex Prentif Cap (see Fig. 1) and the silicone Femcap. Because there are only three (Femcap) or four (Prentif) sizes, it is not possible to find one to fit every woman. Because cervical caps seldom are used, it can be hard to purchase the device or find a practitioner who can fit one. The Internet can be useful in this regard; some useful websites are www.cervcap.com for the Prentif Cap (which lists pharmacies who carry it and locations to get fitted) and www.femcap.com.

Efficacy

The cervical cap is less effective in parous women. Failure rates for nulliparous women are 9% and 16% for perfect and typical use, respectively, which is comparable to the sponge and slightly less effective than the diaphragm. Parous women have a much higher failure rate of 26% for perfect use and 32% for typical use [8,65].

Advantages

The main advantage of the cervical cap is that it can be worn continuously for 48 hours and that extra spermicide is not required for additional acts of coitus during that time. The cervical cap may be associated less with urinary tract infections than the diaphragm because it does not put pressure on the urethra, but the data on this are conflicting [40,66]. The Femcap is nonlatex.

Disadvantages

Some women may find the cervical cap difficult to insert. It is not recommended for use during menstruation because of the theoretical risk of toxic shock syndrome. Oil-based lubricants and vaginal medications must be avoided with the latex Prentif cap. Concerns about cervical dysplasia with the cap largely have been disproven [67].

Tips for proper use and patient counseling

Cervical caps also traditionally are used with spermicidal jelly. The cap is squeezed, inserted into the vagina with the open side up, pushed along the posterior wall of the vagina as far as it can go, and then adjusted to cover the cervix. It stays in place by suction. Like the diaphragm, it can be placed before intercourse, but the cap can be left in place for up to 48 hours, and repeat applications of spermicide are not required for subsequent acts of intercourse. It should be left in place for at least 6 to 8 hours after the last intercourse, depending on the manufacturer's instructions.

Summary

All barrier methods are safe, have essentially no systemic effects, and only need to be used at the time of coitus. The ideal barrier for teenagers continues to be the latex condom for its dual protection and its ease of access and use. Worldwide, latex male condoms are an invaluable strategy in the battle against HIV/AIDS. The female condom provides a nonlatex, woman-controlled alternative for pregnancy and STI prevention, and thus should be mentioned.

Unfortunately, many teenagers lack the comfort and confidence to use one of the more "cumbersome" barrier methods, but for the well-motivated, educated teen this may not be true. A user of any barrier method can combine it with a separately inserted spermicide to improve contraceptive efficacy, especially if pregnancy would be devastating. Likewise, a male condom can be added to a vaginal barrier method (except the female condom), or any contraceptive method. Discussion about emergency contraception should occur when counseling about barrier methods, and a prescription given in advance in case there is a mishap.

Acknowledgments

Thanks to Mr. Chris Peck, Medical Photography Services, Queen's University, Kingston, ON, Canada for his assistance with the photographs.

References

[1] Barrier methods. In: Speroff L, Darney PD, editors. A clinical guide for contraception. 3rd edition. Philadelphia: Lippincott Williams & Wilkins; 2001. p. 259–95.

[2] Condoms. In: Hatcher RA, Trussell J, Stewart F, et al, editors. Contraceptive technology. 16th edition. New York: Irvington Publishers, Inc.; 1994. p. 145–77.

[3] Fisher W, Boroditsky R, Morris B. The 2002 Canadian contraception study: part 1. J Obstet Gynaecol Can 2004;26(6):580–90.

[4] Manhart LE, Koutsky LA. Do condoms prevent genital HPV infection, external genital warts or cervical neoplasia? A meta-analysis. Sex Transm Dis 2002;29(11):725–35.

[5] Weller S, Davis K. Condom effectiveness in reducing heterosexual HIV transmission. Cochrane Database Syst Rev 2005;3:CD003255.

[6] Cates W, Stone KM. Family planning, sexually transmitted diseases and contraceptive choice: a literature update—part 1. Fam Plann Perspect 1992;24(2):75–84.

[7] McNeill ET, Gilmore CE, Finger WR, et al, for Family Health International. The latex condom: recent advances, future directions. Available at: http://www.fhi.org/en/RH/Pubs/booksReports/latexcondom/index.htm. Accessed December 9, 2004.

[8] Trussell J. Contraceptive failure in the United States. Contraception 2004;70:89–96.

[9] Darrow WW. Condom use and use-effectiveness in high-risk populations. Sex Transm Dis 1989;16(3):157–9.

[10] Albert AE, Hatcher RA, Graves W. Condom use and breakage among women in a municipal hospital family planning clinic. Contraception 1991;43(2):167–76.

[11] Trussell J, Warner DL, Hatcher RA. Condom slippage and breakage rates. Fam Plann Perspect 1992;24(1):20–3.

[12] Trussell J, Warner DL, Hatcher RA. Condom performance during vaginal intercourse: comparison of Trojan-Enz and Tactylon condoms. Contraception 1992;45(1):11–9.

[13] Leeper MA, Conrardy M. Preliminary evaluation of REALITY, a condom for women to wear. Adv Contracept 1989;5:229–35.

[14] World Health Organization. WHO/CONRAD technical consultation on nonoxynol-9; summary report. Geneva: WHO; 2001. Available at: http://www.who.int/reproductive-health/rtis/nonoxynol9.html. Accessed November 4, 2004.

[15] Kestelman P, Trussell J. Efficacy of the simultaneous use of condoms and spermicides. Fam Plann Perspect 1991;23(5):226–7, 232.

[16] Voeller B, Coulson AH, Bernstein GS, et al. Mineral oil lubricants cause rapid deterioration of latex condoms. Contraception 1989;39(1):95–102.

[17] Drew WL, Blair M, Miner RC, et al. Evaluation of the virus permeability of a new condom for women. Sex Transm Dis 1990;17(2):110–2.

[18] Voeller B, Coulter SL, Mayhan KG. Gas, dye and viral transport through polyurethane condoms. JAMA 1991;266(21):2986–7.

[19] Frezieres RG, Walsh TL, Nelson AL, et al. Evaluation of the efficacy of a polyurethane condom: results from a randomized, controlled clinical trial. Fam Plann Perspect 1999;31(2):81–7.

[20] Gallo MF, Grimes DA, Schulz KF. Non-latex versus latex male condoms for contraception. Cochrane Database Syst Rev 2005;(3):CD003550.

[21] Steiner MJ, Dominik R, Rountree RW, et al. Contraceptive effectiveness of a polyurethane condom and a latex condom: a randomized controlled trial. Obstet Gynecol 2003;101(3):539–47.

[22] Cook L, Nanda K, Taylor D. Randomized crossover trial comparing the eZ.on plastic condom and a latex condom. Contraception 2001;63:25–31.

[23] Callahan M, Mauck C, Taylor D, et al. Comparative evaluation of three Tactylon condoms and a latex condom during vaginal intercourse: breakage and slippage. Contraception 2000; 61:205–15.

[24] Planned Parenthood Federation of America, Inc. Birth control; over-the-counter barrier methods. Available at: http://www.plannedparenthood.org/bc/cchoices5.html#OVERTHECOUNTER. Accessed November 27, 2004.

[25] Farr G, Gabelnick H, Sturgen K, et al. Contraceptive efficacy and acceptability of the female condom. Am J Public Health 1994;84(12):1960–4.

[26] Trussell J, Sturgen K, Strickler J, et al. Comparative contraceptive efficacy of the female condom and other barrier methods. Fam Plann Perspect 1994;26(2):66–72.

[27] Bounds W, Guillebaud J, Newman GB. Female condom (Femidom). A clinical study of its use-effectiveness and patient acceptability. Br J Fam Plann 1992;18(2):36–41.

[28] Trussell J. Contraceptive efficacy of the Reality female condom. Contraception 1998;58:147–8.

[29] French PP, Latka M, Gollub EL, et al. Use-effectiveness of the female versus male condom in preventing sexually transmitted disease in women. Sex Transm Dis 2003;30(5):433–9.

[30] International Planned Parenthood Federation. IMAP statement on barrier methods of contraception. IPPF Med Bull 2001;35(4):1–2.

[31] Soper DE, Shoupe D, Shangold GA, et al. Prevention of vaginal trichomoniasis by compliant use of the female condom. Sex Transm Dis 1993;20(3):137–9.

[32] Family Health International. FHI Research briefs on the female condom—No. 2: effectiveness for preventing pregnancy and sexually transmitted infections. Available at: http://www.fhi. org/en/RH/Pubs/Briefs/fcbriefs/EffectiveSTIs.htm. Accessed November 4, 2004.

[33] The diaphragm, contraceptive sponge, cervical cap & female condom. In: Hatcher RA, Trussell J, Stewart F, et al, editors. Contraceptive technology. 16th edition. New York: Irvington Publishers, Inc.; 1994. p. 191–221.

[34] Fontanet A, Saba J, Chandelying V, et al. Protection against sexually transmitted diseases by granting sex workers in Thailand the choice of using the male or female condom: results from a randomized controlled trial. AIDS 1998;12(14):1851–9.

[35] Jivasak-Apimas S, Saba J, Chandelying V, et al. Acceptability of the female condom among sex workers in Thailand: results from a prospective study. Sex Transm Dis 2001;28(11):648–54.

[36] Family Health International. Technical update on the female condom. Washington (DC): FHI; 2001. Available at: http://www.fhi.org/en/RH/Pubs/booksReports/fcupdate.htm. Accessed November 4, 2004.

[37] The Female Health Company. FC Female Condom. Available at: http://www.femalehealth.com/theproduct.html. Accessed December 11, 2004.

[38] Family Health International. How effective are spermicides? Network 2000;20(2). Available at: http://www.fhi.org/en/RH/Pubs/Network/v20_2/NWvol20-2spermicids.htm. Accessed December 12, 2004.

[39] Raymond E, Dominik R. Contraceptive effectiveness of two spermicides: a randomized trial. Obstet Gynecol 1999;93(6):896–903.

[40] Hooton TM, Scholes D, Hughes JP, et al. A prospective study of risk factors for symptomatic urinary tract infection in young women. N Engl J Med 1996;335(7):468–74.
[41] Hooton TM, Fennell CL, Clark AM, et al. Nonoxynol-9: differential antibacterial activity and enhancement of bacterial adherence to vaginal epithelial cells. J Infect Dis 1991;164:1216–9.
[42] Hooton TM, Roberts PL, Stamm WE. Effects of recent sexual activity and use of a diaphragm on the vaginal microflora. Clin Infect Dis 1994;19:274–8.
[43] Hooton TM, Hillier S, Johnson C, et al. *Escherichia coli* bacteriuria and contraceptive method. JAMA 1991;265(1):64–9.
[44] Roddy RE, Zekeng L, Ryan KA, et al. A controlled trial of nonoxynol-9 film to reduce male-to-female transmission of sexually transmitted diseases. N Engl J Med 1998;339(8):504–10.
[45] Van Damme L, Ramjee G, Alary M, et al. Effectiveness of COL-1492, a nonoxynol-9 vaginal gel, on HIV-1 transmission in female sex workers: a randomized controlled trial. Lancet 2002;360:971–7.
[46] Kreiss J, Ngugi E, Holmes K, et al. Efficacy of nonoxynol-9 contraceptive sponge use in preventing heterosexual acquisition of HIV in Nairobi prostitutes. JAMA 1992;268(4):477–82.
[47] Wilkinson D, Ramjee G, Tholandi M, et al. Nonoxynol-9 for preventing vaginal acquisition of HIV infection by women from men. Cochrane Database Syst Rev 2002;(3):CD 003936.
[48] Wilkinson D, Ramjee G, Tholandi M, et al. Nonoxynol-9 for preventing vaginal acquisition of sexually transmitted infections by women from men. Cochrane Database Syst Rev 2002;(1): CD 003939.
[49] Sangi-Haghpeykar H, Poindexter AN, Levine H. Sperm transport and survival post-application of a new spermicide contraceptive. Advantage 24 Study Group. Contraception 1996;53:353–6.
[50] Kuyoh MA, Toroitich-Ruto C, Grimes DA, et al. Sponge versus diaphragm for contraception: a Cochrane review. Contraception 2003;67:15–8.
[51] Birthcontrol.com. Available at: http://www.birthcontrol.com. Accessed July 5, 2005.
[52] McIntyre SL, Higgins J. Parity and use-effectiveness with the contraceptive sponge. Am J Obstet Gynecol 1986;155(4):796–801.
[53] Creatsas G, Guerrero E, Guilbert E, et al. A multinational evaluation of the efficacy, safety and acceptability of the Protectaid contraceptive sponge. Eur J Contracept Reprod Health Care 2001;6(3):172–82.
[54] Faich G, Pearson K, Fleming D, et al. Toxic shock syndrome and the vaginal contraceptive sponge. JAMA 1986;255(2):216–8.
[55] Francoeur D, Hanvey L, Miller R, et al. In: Barrier methods. Black A, Francoeur D, Rowe T, editors. Canadian Contraception Consensus. J Obstet Gynaecol Can 2004;26(4):347–63.
[56] Milex Products, Inc. Wide Seal silicone diaphragms. Available at: http://www.milexproducts. com/products/other/diaphrams.asp. Accessed December 12, 2004.
[57] Smith C, Farr G, Feldblum PJ, et al. Effectiveness of the non-spermicidal fit-free diaphragm. Contraception 1995;51:289–91.
[58] Bounds W, Guillebaud J, Dominik R, et al. The diaphragm with and without spermicide: a randomized, comparative efficacy trial. J Reprod Med 1995;40(11):764–74.
[59] Cook L, Nanda K, Grimes D. Diaphragm versus diaphragm with spermicides for contraception. Cochrane Database Syst Rev 2003;(1):CD002031.
[60] Family Health International. Will diaphragms protect against STIs? Network 2003;22(4). Available at: http://www.fhi.org/en/RH/Pubs/Network/v22_4/nt2246.htm. Accessed December 12, 2004.
[61] Fisher M, Marks A, Trieller K. Comparative analysis of the effectiveness of the diaphragm and birth control pill during the first year of use among suburban adolescents. J Adolesc Health Care 1987;8(5):393–9.
[62] Lane ME, Arceo R, Sobrero AJ. Successful use of the diaphragm and jelly by a young population: report of a clinical study. Fam Plann Perspect 1976;8(2):81–6.
[63] Mauck C, Glover LH, Miller E, et al. Lea's Shield: a study of the safety and efficacy of a new vaginal barrier contraceptive used with and without spermicide. Contraception 1996;53:329–35.
[64] United States Food and Drug Administration. Summary of safety and effectiveness data on Lea's Sheild. Available at: http://www.fda.gov/cdrh/pdf/P010043b.pdf. Accessed December 12, 2004.

[65] Trussell J, Strickler J, Vaughan B. Contraceptive efficacy of the diaphragm, the sponge and the cervical cap. Fam Plann Perspect 1993;25(3):100–5, 135.

[66] Gallo MF, Grimes DA, Schulz KF. Cervical cap versus diaphragm for contraception. Cochrane Database Syst Rev 2002;(4):CD003551.

[67] Gollub EL, Sivin I. The Prentif cervical cap and pap smear results: a critical appraisal. Contraception 1989;40(3):343–9.

ELSEVIER
SAUNDERS

ADOLESCENT
MEDICINE
CLINICS

Adolesc Med 16 (2005) 517–537

Combined Hormonal Contraception

Michele E. Calderoni, DO*, Susan M. Coupey, MD

*Section of Adolescent Medicine, Children's Hospital at Montefiore/Albert Einstein College of Medicine,
111 East 210th Street, Bronx, NY 10467, USA*

Adolescents in the United States have more contraceptive options available to them today then ever before. The pregnancy rate among 15- to 17-year-old girls declined 33% between 1991 and 2000; yet, effective contraceptive use by US teens continues to be a problem [1]. In 2001, 13% of sexually active 15- to 17-year olds used no method of contraception at last intercourse. In 2000, more than 300,000 adolescents became pregnant, and 166,000 adolescents gave birth [1,2]. Associations between early adolescent parenting and adverse social and health consequences for mother and child have been established [3].

At the same time as the teen pregnancy rate in the United States has been declining, the use of hormonal contraception also has been declining, while condom use has increased. There are many barriers facing adolescents who wish to use hormonal contraceptives, including issues of confidentiality, cost, access, and misperceptions of adverse effects. A comprehensive analysis of peer-reviewed articles between 1980 and 2000 reported that many adolescents believe that hormonal contraceptives cause serious adverse health consequences such as permanent infertility, cancer, and birth defects [4]. Clinicians providing contraceptive counseling to adolescents have the opportunity to address the obstacles and dispel the myths and misperceptions that many teens believe.

Historical perspective

The US Food and Drug Administration (FDA) approved the first oral contraceptive, Norethynodrel, in 1960 [5]. The hormonal formulation of Enovid was 150 µg of mestranol (equivalent to 120 µg of ethinyl estradiol) [6] and 9.85 mg of

* Corresponding author.
E-mail address: mcaldero@montefiore.org (M.E. Calderoni).

1547-3368/05/$ – see front matter © 2005 Elsevier Inc. All rights reserved.
doi:10.1016/j.admecli.2005.05.001

norethynodrel and provided a much higher dose of both the estrogen and pro-gestin components than pills used today. The high hormonal doses made these first OCPs difficult to tolerate, with a narrow safety profile [6]. High-dose estro-gen OCPs have been shown to be associated with an increased risk of myocardial infarction (MI), cerebral vascular accidents (CVA), and venous thromboembo-lism (VTE) [7]. Changes in coagulation and fibrinolysis variables favoring hy-percoagulability are seen with OCPs containing as low a dose as 50 μg ethinyl estradiol (EE). Meade and colleagues demonstrated a lower incidence of death and ischemic heart disease with a 30 μg dose of EE as compared with a 50 μg dose of EE [8]. Other studies have shown a higher relative risk (RR) of CVA and VTE with high doses of EE (at least 50 μg) as compared with that seen in OCPs with less than 50 μg of EE [9–11]. In light of this evidence, OCPs in general use for contraception today are termed "low-dose" and contain 35 μg of EE or less. Additionally, there have been no reports of increased rates of MI and no attrib-utable risk of death from cardiovascular disease related to use of OCPs con-taining less than 50 μg of EE in adolescents [12–14].

Use of OCPs with low doses of estrogen also has decreased the rate of less serious adverse effects such as headaches, breast tenderness, nausea, and weight gain [15].

More recently, attention has turned to improving the adverse effect profile of the progestational component of OCPs. In the 1990s, the FDA approved two new progestational agents, norgestimate and desogestrel, as components of low-dose combination pills. These third generation progestins are more selective for the progesterone receptor and have less affinity for the androgen receptor than first-and second-generation progestins. Thus, combination pills containing these pro-gestins may have fewer androgenic adverse effects such as acne, hair loss, and atherogenic lipid changes. Indeed, the FDA recently approved one third-generation progestin pill, Norgestimate, for treatment of acne, the first approved noncontraceptive indication for an OCP. In 2001, an OCP (Drospirenone) with a progestin from a completely different family, drospirenone, an analog of spi-ronolactone, was approved for use in the United States. This progestin has antiandrogenic activity and theoretically further reduces the androgenic adverse effects of synthetic progestins in OCPs.

The evolution of the pharmacological profile of OCPs over the past 40 years allows women to enjoy the benefits of an effective, reversible contraceptive method with diminished hormone-related adverse effects. Along with improve-ments in the dose and type of hormones, changes have been made in the delivery of these combined hormone formulations, with the aim of increasing adherence and decreasing the rate of unintended pregnancies.

Oral contraceptive pills

Oral contraceptive pills are the most widely used form of combined hormonal contraception by adolescents in the United States [1,16]. OCPs most often are used by teens as a convenient method of birth control that is safe, effective, reversible, and does not interfere with sexual spontaneity. OCPs also offer many therapeutic and noncontraceptive health benefits and often also are used by adolescents to treat medical conditions such as dysfunctional uterine bleeding, endometriosis and functional ovarian hyperandrogenism.

Combined hormonal OCPs are packaged in 21- or 28-day cycles. The 21-day cycle pack includes 21 active pills with no placebo pills in the pack. Whereas the 28-day cycle pack includes 21 active pills and 7 placebo pills and may encourage better adherence and ease of use, especially for adolescents. Table 1 lists selected OCPs with their hormonal content. OCPs are categorized into monophasic or triphasic formulations. The monophasic pill pack has 21 active pills with the same dose of hormones (EE and a progestin) in each pill. Triphasic OCPs have differing amounts of either the EE or the progestin or both throughout the cycle.

Overview of mechanism of action

The mechanism of action of OCPs has not changed over the years despite pharmacological changes. OCPs act on four distinct areas, all of which contribute to the efficacy of this method. The estrogen and progestin components inhibit ovulation by interfering with the hypothalamic-pituitary-ovarian (HPO) axis. Estrogen and progestin inhibit ovulation through negative feedback on the HPO axis and suppress follicle stimulating hormone (FSH) secretion and the surge of luteinizing hormone (LH) secretion that triggers ovulation [17]. Both hormones in combined OCPs also alter the lining of the endometrium, making implantation

Table 1
Formulation profiles of selected oral contraceptive pills

Type	Brand name	Ethinyl estradiol (μg/d)	Type of progestin	Progestin (mg/d)
Monophasic	Alesse	20	Levonorgestrel	0.1
	Loestrin 1/20	20	Norethindrone acetate	1
	Ortho-Cept	30	Desogestrel	0.15
	Lo/Ovral	30	Norgestrel	0.3
	Nordette	30	Levonorgestrel	0.15
	Ortho-Cyclen	35	Norgestimate	0.25
	Ortho-Novum 1/35	35	Norethindrone	1
	Yasmin	30	Drospirenone	3
Triphasic	Ortho Tri-Cyclen	35	Norgestimate	0.18 × 7 d
				0.215 × 7d
				0.25 × 7 d
	Triphasil	30 × 7 d	Levonorgestrel	0.05 × 7 d
		40 × 7 d		0.075 × 7 d
		30 × 7d		0.125 × 7 d
Extended 91-day cycle	Seasonale	30	Levonorgestrel	0.15

of a fertilized ovum less likely [17]. The progestin component of the OCP thickens the cervical mucus, making it difficult for sperm to enter into the uterus and fallopian tubes, where fertilization usually occurs [17]. Progestin also reduces the activity of the cilia in the fallopian tubes, decreasing tubal transport [17].

Pharmacology

Estrogen

Oral contraceptive pills are a combination of orally active synthetic forms of estrogen and progesterone. There is a daily peak and trough in hormone concentration with OCPs, and they should be taken approximately every 24 hours, at the same time every day [18]. Because OCPs are taken by mouth, they undergo first-pass metabolism in the liver, thus requiring higher doses of hormones as compared with other routes of administration to ensure therapeutic drug levels in the blood stream [18]. All combined hormonal OCPs use EE; however, the dose ranges from 20 35 μg EE per pill. The selection of one dose of EE over another is predicated on the estrogen-related adverse effects the user experiences.

Poindexter evaluated over 150 articles to study the efficacy, safety, and tolerability of 20 μg EE OCPs [7]. In his review, he found that OCPs with 20 μg EE had a contraceptive efficacy rate, as measured by the Pearl Index, in the range of 0.07 to 2.1, which compares favorably with OCPs with EE doses of 30 μg and 35 μg. Other factors that were evaluated by this review were cycle control (spotting and breakthrough bleeding), safety, and noncontraceptive health benefits of OCPs. Adequate cycle control is an important factor in determining compliance. If problematic, lack of cycle control can be the single most important reason for OCP discontinuation [19,20]. When evaluating cycle control with the 20 μg EE formulation, it is also important to note the type of progestin included in the OCP. Studies suggest that the type of progestin can influence cycle control [7]. Pills containing a 20 μg dose of EE with a gonane progestin (eg, levonorgestrel/norgestimate) appear to have better cycle control than those with an estrane progestin (eg, norethindrone acetate) [7].

Relative to safety concerns, Poindexter reported that 20 μg and 30 μg EE OCP formulations have similar hemostatic effects [7]. There are limited data on the effects of 20 μg EE OCPs on lipid parameters; however, they may have a more favorable profile than OCPs with 30 μg of EE, as seen by small increases in serum high-density lipoprotein (HDL) and small decreases in serum low-density lipoprotein (LDL) with the 20 μg pills [21,22]. It is unknown, however, whether these small changes are clinically significant. Studies have demonstrated a lower discontinuation rate with 20 μg OCPs than with 30 μg and 35 μg OCPs, presumably because of fewer estrogen-related adverse effects [23–25].

It is important to note that no specific OCP formulation has been shown to reduce the incidence of estrogen-related adverse effects consistently. The 20 μg estrogen OCPs, however, may be beneficial in individual patients. Over time, this may translate into improved user satisfaction and continuation rates.

Progestin

There are three categories of synthetic progestins that have been used in OCPs: estranes, gonanes, and drospirenone [26]. Estranes were used in the first OCPs in the 1960s and 1970s. These progestins are a homogenous chemical family and include norethynodrel, norethindrone, and norethindrone acetate. Conversion to norethindrone must occur for estranes to become biologically active [26]. Gonanes are more potent progestins, and many are chemically distinct, giving them a different biological profile [26]. The prototypical gonane progestin is levonorgestrel (LNG), the active isomer of norgestrel. In the 1980s, three high-potency gonane progestins, often termed third-generation progestins, were developed: norgestimate (NGM), desogestrel (DSG), and gestodene (GSD) [6]. Norgestimate and desogestrel are available for clinical use worldwide, but gestodene is not approved for use in the United States. These newer gonanes were developed in an attempt to minimize androgenic effects while delivering equivalent progestational potency as the older progestins [27].

Synthetic progestins work by binding to both progesterone and androgen receptors. The ratio of a progestin's ability to bind to these receptors is expressed as the androgen-to-progesterone binding ratio [27]. The higher the ratio, the greater the difference between progestional (desired) and androgenic (undesired) responses. The gonane NGM has a low androgen binding affinity in vitro, whereas LNG has one of the highest [28,29]. The difference between the two properties suggests that NGM may produce fewer androgenic adverse effects such as hirsutism and acne as compared with LNG [27]. In addition to exerting a direct androgenic effect by binding to androgen receptors, progestins also may produce an indirect androgenic response by their effect on sex hormone binding globulin (SHBG) [26]. Studies have shown that NGM has almost no binding affinity for SBHG in vitro [26]. In contrast, LNG has a relatively high binding affinity for SHBG and may displace endogenous androgen, mainly testosterone, thus rendering it biologically active [26]. Therefore, a combined hormonal OCP with NGM may be a better option for a user with acne, hirsutism, or functional ovarian hyperandrogenism as compared with other progestins used in OCPs. It must be stressed, however, that the overall androgenicity effect of a specific OCP on an individual patient is dependent on a multitude of host and pill factors and cannot be predicted solely from in vitro studies.

Additionally, some progestins have an inhibitory effect on the enzyme 5-alpha reductase, which converts testosterone to dihydrotestosterone, the active androgen in skin and hair follicles [30]. Clinically, this property should improve acne and hirsutism. Of the progestins studied, NGM was the most powerful 5-alpha reductase inhibitor, followed by LNG [30].

Efficacy

When discussing efficacy rates in OCP use, most studies refer to typical use versus perfect use when reporting probabilities of pregnancy within the first year of method use. Typical use reflects how effective the method is for an average person who may or may not always use the method correctly or consistently. This can be quite variable, as it pertains to the user's perception of what using a method actually means. Perfect use implies that the method was used correctly and consistently with every act of sexual intercourse [31]. Other studies use the term Pearl Index, which is defined as the number of pregnancies per 100 woman-years of treatment [7]. Trussell reviewed more than 165 articles on contraceptive failure and found that for typical OCP users, 8% of women experience an unintended pregnancy during the first year. For perfect OCP users, the rate decreased substantially to 0.3% [31].

Adverse events

Adverse effects from OCP use are categorized as estrogen-related, progesterone-related, or androgen-related. Estrogen-related adverse effects include nausea, fluid retention, headaches, breast tenderness, breakthrough bleeding and spotting, and hypertension. Using a 20 μg EE formulation may help alleviate these adverse effects if they occur [15]. Progesterone-related adverse effects include menstrual changes, fatigue, and depression [32–34]. Androgen-related adverse effects include oily hair and skin, hirsutism, male-pattern hair loss, increased appetite with weight gain, and acne. Using OCPs with less androgenic progestins may help to alleviate these effects.

Studies in adult women have demonstrated a small increase in the relative risk of localized breast cancer associated with current OCP use, (RR 1.24; 95% confidence interval [CI], 1.15 to 1.33) as compared with controls [35]. The risk was shown to decline shortly after discontinuation and disappears within 10 years. The incidence of MI and CVA are very rare among young, healthy reproductive-age women. Epidemiologic studies have demonstrated that the use of OCPs does not increase the risk of MI or CVA in nonsmoking women of reproductive age who have no pre-existing cardiovascular disease [12,36–38]. An analysis of 220 articles that studied the relationship between OCP use and VTE estimated the baseline rate of deep vein thrombosis to be 5 to 10 events per 100,000 nonpregnant reproductive age women [39]. The use of OCPs in this population increases the risk of VTE to 10 to 30 events per 100,000 users [39]. This increase, however, is still much less than the risk of VTE in pregnancy. In terms of lipid parameters, the estrogen dose and the androgenicity of the progestin determine the effect. The estrogen component increases triglycerides and HDL and decreases serum LDL [40]. Androgenic progestins increase LDL and lower HDL [40]. Progestins such as norgestimate, desogestrel, and drospirenone (low or no androgen affinity binding effect) actually raise HDL and lower LDL [40–43].

Contraindications

Medical contraindications to OCPs are based on the World Health Organization's (WHO's) recommendations to help guide health care providers when prescribing OCPs to women with medical conditions [44]. The WHO has developed four medical eligibility classification categories based on a risk/benefit ratio (the risk of the interaction of the hormonal contraception with the specific medical condition versus the benefits of the OCP). These same guidelines can be applied to adolescents. Category One lists medical conditions for which there are no restrictions to OCP use. Examples include benign breast disease and epilepsy. Category Two includes medical conditions for which the advantages of using OCPs outweigh the theoretical or proven risks. Conditions such as diabetes mellitus and sickle cell disease are examples. Medical conditions included under Category Three are those in which the theoretical or proven risk usually outweighs the advantages of using OCPs. If OCPs are used in women with these medical conditions, close monitoring is advised. Examples of such conditions include gallbladder disease and women who are postpartum less than 21 days. Category Four lists medical conditions that are contraindications to using OCPs. This includes current or history of VTE, current liver disease, and headaches with neurological symptoms. For a complete list of medical conditions by each category refer to Table 2 [44].

Advantages

Oral contraceptive pills offer many noncontraceptive benefits to the adolescent user. These include improvement of dysmenorrhea, acne, bone mineral density, functional ovarian hyperandrogenism, cycle control, and suppression of ovarian and benign breast cyst formation. Additionally, OCPs have been shown to decrease the risk of endometrial, ovarian, and colorectal cancers, and to lower the risk of pelvic inflammatory disease. These are discussed in more detail in the article by Hatim Omar elsewhere in this issue [45,46].

In addition to the noncontraceptive benefits, OCPs can be an excellent method of contraception for an adolescent. The method is safe, well tolerated, and reversible. There are many formulations, thus enabling health care providers to choose an OCP that best serves the clinical profile of the adolescent.

Numerous professional organizations, including WHO, the American College of Obstetricians and Gynecologists, and the Society of Adolescent Medicine, have stated that a gynecological examination is not necessary to initiate OCP treatment. All agree that sexually active adolescents should have an annual pelvic examination to screen for sexually transmitted infections (STIs) and cervical cancer, but this should not be a prerequisite to prescribing OCPs.

Disadvantages

The daily dosing schedule of OCPs may be a barrier to perfect use and may result in unintended pregnancies. A review of over 1000 OCP users in the 1995 National Survey of Family Growth found that 16% of sexually active users were inconsistent pill takers [47]. Studies evaluating inconsistent pill use found that adolescents miss an average of three pills per month, and at least 20% to 30% of adolescents miss a pill every month [48]. Adolescent OCP users who missed one

Table 2
Medical eligibility criteria for combined hormonal contraceptive use

Medical condition	Category	Comments
Pregnancy	NA	There is no known harm to the woman, pregnancy, or fetus if OCPs are used accidentally during pregnancy
Age		
Menarche to <40	1	
≥40	2	
Parity		
Nulliparous	1	
Parous	1	
Breastfeeding		
<6 wks postpartum	4	Theoretical risk of infant exposure to steroids and risk of thrombosis in mother
≥6 wks to <6 months	3	In first 6 months, OCPs may decrease quantity of breast milk.
>6 months	2	
Post partum		
In non breastfeeding women		
<21 days	3	Blood coagulation and fibrinolysis are normalized by 3 wks postpartum.
≥21 days	1	
Post abortion	1	OCPs may be started immediately after a termination regardless of trimester.
Smoking		
<35 years	2	
>35 years	3	
Obesity (body mass index of >30)	2	Obesity is a risk factor for venous thromboembolism.
Cardiovascular conditions		
Hypertension		
Controlled	3	
Not controlled	3–4	
Deep venous thrombosis/pulmonary embolus (DVT/PE)		
History of DVT/PE	4	
Current DVT/PE	4	
First-degree relative with DVT/PE	2	Consider screening for heritable coagulopathy.
Major surgery		
Prolonged immobilization	4	
Without prolonged immobilization	2	
Superficial venous Thrombosis		
Varicose veins	1	
Superficial thrombophlebitis	2	
Current and history of ischemic heart disease	4	Women with underlying vascular disease should avoid OCPs.
Cerebral vascular accident	4	
Hyperlipidemias	2–3	The category should be assessed according to type of lipidemia and the presence of other cardiovascular risk factors.

Table 2 (*continued*)

Medical condition	Category	Comments
Valvular heart disease		
Uncomplicated	2	
Complicated[a]	4	
Neurologic conditions		
Headaches		
Nonmigrainous	1–2	
Migraine		
Without neurologic symptoms	2–3	Over the age of 35 the category changes to 3–4.
With neurologic symptoms	4	
Seizures	1	Check interactions of antiepileptic with OCPs.
Reproductive tract conditions		
Irregular bleeding patterns	1–2	There are no conditions that cause vaginal bleeding that will be worsened in the short term by the use of OCPs.
Endometriosis	1	May alleviate symptoms.
Benign ovarian tumors and cysts	1	
Dysmenorrhea	1	May alleviate symptoms.
Cervical ectropion	1	
Trophoblastic disease	1	
Cervical intraepithelial neoplasm	2	OCPs may enhance progression to invasive disease with long-term use.
Breast disease		
Undiagnosed mass	2	
Benign breast disease	1	
Family history of breast cancer	1	
History of breast cancer		
Current	4	
Past	3	
Endometrial cancer	1	OCP use reduces the risk of endometrial cancer; a women may use OCPs while awaiting therapy.
Ovarian cancer	1	OCP use reduces the risk of ovarian cancer; women may use OCPs while awaiting therapy.
Uterine fibroids	1	
Pelvic inflammatory disease	1	OCPs may reduce the risk of sexually transmitted infections (STIs).
STIs	1	
HIV/AIDS	1	
Endocrine conditions		
Diabetes		
Gestational	1	
Nonvascular	2	
Vascular complications[b]	3–4	Assess category according to the severity of the condition.
Thyroid disorders		
All conditions	1	

(continued on next page)

Table 2 (*continued*)

Medical condition	Category	Comments
Gastrointestinal disorders		
Gallbladder disease		
Symptomatic		
Cholecystectomy	2	OCPs may cause or worsen gall bladder disease.
Medically treated	3	
Current	3	
Asymptomatic	2	
History of cholestasis		
Related to pregnancy	2	
Related to OCP use	3	
Viral hepatitis		
Active	4	
Carrier	1	
Cirrhosis		
Mild (compensated)	3	
Severe (decompensated)	4	
Liver tumors		
Benign or malignant	4	
Hematologic conditions		
Thalassaemia	1	
Sickle cell	2	
Fe defiency anemia	1	

[a] Refers to Pulmonary hypertension, atrial fibrillation, history of subacute bacterial endocarditis.
[b] Includes nephropathy, retinopathy, neuropathy.
Adapted from the World Health Organization.

or more pills per month were found to be three times as likely to become pregnant as compared with adolescents who took their pills consistently [32].

Irregular bleeding such as breakthrough bleeding, spotting, or amenorrhea frequently causes adolescents to discontinue OCP use [49]. Poor cycle control has been found to make young women less confident about the OCP and the health care provider [49]. Irregular bleeding with OCPs has been shown to increase health care provider visits and anxiety about potential pregnancy. Over time, this can lead to poor adherence or discontinuation [49].

Another disadvantage of OCPs, particularly relevant for adolescents, is cost. A 1-month supply of OCPs costs approximately $35. Many adolescents cannot depend on their parents' insurance or income to pay for OCPs; therefore they must pay for the pills themselves. Furthermore, if the OCP use is confidential, concealing pill packs from parents and guardians may be challenging. Confidentiality also may be compromised if adolescents use the same community/local pharmacies as their parents; the pharmacist may inadvertently give filled prescriptions to parents or family members.

Another disadvantage is that to use this method an adolescent must seek a visit from a health care provider to obtain a prescription. Here too, issues such as confidentiality and cost may act as barriers.

New oral contraceptive pills

Yasmin

In 2001, the FDA approved a new OCP, marketed under the name Yasmin. This is the first OCP containing the progestin drospirenone, an analog of spironolactone. What makes this progestin unique is its antiandrogen and anti-mineralcorticoid properties. Drospirenone was shown in animal models to more closely resemble the pharmacological properties of natural progesterone as compared with other synthetic progestins [50]. Yasmin contains 3 mg of drospirenone and 30 μg EE [43]. In an open-label, multi-center study, Parsey and colleagues evaluated 333 women, aged 18 to 35 years, and demonstrated that Yasmin's contraceptive effectiveness, as measured by the Pearl Index, was similar to that of other combination OCPs, 0.406 versus 0 to 1, respectively [43,51]. They also showed that this new combination OCP had acceptable cycle control rates that were similar to those seen with published studies of other OCPs. Additionally, Yasmin had a favorable profile with respect to weight, lipids, and blood pressure. From her findings, Paresy also suggested that this unique progestin/EE combination may decrease the severity of some menstrual and premenstrual symptoms [43]. The antiandrogenic properties of drospirenone make Yasmin a good OCP choice for adolescents with functional ovarian hyperandrogenism. Because of its antimineralcorticoid properties, Yasmin should not be used by adolescents at risk for hyperkalemia. This includes teens with medical conditions such as renal insufficiency, hepatic insufficiency, adrenal insufficiency, and those on angiotensin-converting enzyme inhibitors, angiotensin II receptor antagonists, and nonsteroidal anti-inflammatory drugs [52].

Seasonale

Approved by the FDA in 2003, Seasonale is a new contraceptive method packaged as a 91-day extended combined hormonal OCP, with 84 days of hormones and 7 days of placebo. This method gives the user four menstrual periods a year. Seasonal has 30 μg EE and 150 μg LNG.

Anderson and colleagues performed the first large-scale study evaluating the efficacy and safety of Seasonale [53]. The study was a randomized, multi-center, open-label, 1-year evaluation comparing Seasonale with a combined 28-day OCP, Nordette-28 (30 μg EE 150 μg LNG). The safety profile and tolerability were found to be similar. Efficacy rates, using the Pearl index calculations based on method failure, were found to be 0.60 and 1.78 for Seasonale and Nordette-28, respectively. In addition, no pregnancies occurred in women weighing over 90 kg. The Seasonale users did report slightly higher rates of breakthrough bleeding and spotting as compared with the Nordette-28 users, 3.6% days (out of a total of 336 active therapy days) on the extended cycle versus 2.9% days (out of a total of 273 days) on the 28-day cycle. The amount of breakthrough bleeding and spotting in the extended cycle group, however, decreased with each successive cycle, and by the end of the study, the incidence of bleeding was similar between the two groups [53].

Other studies have demonstrated advantages to continuous cycling such as decreasing dysmenorrhea, bloating, mastalgia, menstrual migraine, and iron deficiency anemia from menorrmetrohagia [54].

Newer methods of delivery

Since OCPs were first introduced in the 1960s, the pharmacology has changed so that newer pill regimens are safer, have fewer adverse effects, and have better compliance rates. It has been documented that OCPs remain the most common form of hormonal birth control used by adolescents [1,16]. Despite the improvements in the pill over the past 40 years, however, epidemiological studies suggest typical use of OCPs by adolescent girls produces a failure rate between 5% and 18% [1,7,55,56]. Data from the 1995 National Survey of Family Growth shows that only 58% of adolescents 15 to 17 years of age report perfect compliance with OCPs [16]. Poor compliance, in addition to method failure, or discontinuation without substitution of another effective method, can result in unintended pregnancies.

Recently, new delivery systems have been developed to provide alternate forms of reversible hormonal contraception with similar efficacy, tolerability, and safety characteristics of the well-established OCP. Most importantly, the newer delivery systems are intended to improve adherence and overall user satisfaction and decrease the high rate of unintended adolescent pregnancies. Currently, the newest combined hormonal options include a transdermal patch, a vaginal ring, and a monthly injection that is no longer available. Table 3 illustrates comparisons between OCPs, the transdermal patch, and the vaginal ring.

Transdermal combined hormonal system

The FDA approved the OrthoEvra patch in 2002, and it is the only transdermal combined hormonal system available for use. The patch is beige and measures 4×5 cm (20 cm^2). It consists of three layers: an outer protective layer of polyester, a medicated adhesive middle layer, and a clear polyester release liner that is removed before patch application [57]. The patch can be applied to the buttocks, upper outer arm, lower abdomen or upper torso (excluding the breasts). All sites have been shown to be equally effective [58]. The patch is worn for 1 week at a time, and is replaced on the same day of each week, for three consecutive weeks followed by a patch-free week to allow for a menstrual period. New patches should not be applied to the same site as the preceding patch. While wearing the patch, adolescents are able to continue activities such as exercising, swimming, and bathing without detachment. The use of oils, creams, or cosmetics around the area of the patch, however, should be discouraged. If a patch does not adhere for the entire week, it should be replaced with a new patch immediately. The replacement patch is worn for the remainder of the week and should be changed on the patch change day.

Table 3
Comparison of combined hormonal contraceptive methods

Method	Monthly cost ($)	Efficacy	Type of progestin	EE[a] μg/day	Prescription needed	Reversible	Dosing	Advantages	Disadvantages
OCPs	20–50	99%	Levonorgestrel, norethindrone acetate, norgestrel, desogestrel, norgestimate, norethindrone, drospirenone	20, 30, 35	Yes	Yes	Daily	Discreet; efficacious; non-contraceptive benefits; multiple formulations	Daily dosing; BTB[b]/spotting in first three cycles; estrogen and progestin-related adverse effects
Transdermal patch	36	99%	Norgestromin (metabolized to norgestrel)	20	Yes	Yes	Weekly	Efficacious; weekly dosing; Non-contraceptive benefits[c]	Visible, BTB[b]/spotting in first three cycles; estrogen- and progestin-related adverse effects
Vaginal ring	43	99%	Etonogestrel (metabolized to desogestrel)	15	Yes	Yes	Monthly	Discreet; efficacious; monthly dosing; non-contraceptive benefits[c]	Device-related adverse effects: coital sensation, vaginitis/leukorrhea; self-insertion; estrogen- and progestin-related adverse effects

[a] Ethinyl estradiol.
[b] Breakthrough bleeding.
[c] Noncontraceptive benefits presumed to be similar to OCPs.

In the first published study comparing the patch with OCPs, Audet and colleagues evaluated 811 patch users and found that 4.6% reported complete (1.8%) or partial patch detachment (2.8%) [57]. Adolescent patch users may have a higher rate of detachment (up to 35%), however, as was found by Rubenstein and colleagues in their study of teenage users [59].

Pharmacology

The patch delivers 150 μg of norelgestromin, the primary active metabolite of norgestimate, and 20 μg of ethinyl estradiol daily [60]. The estrogen and progestin components are similar to OCPs, and therefore, the mechanism of action in preventing pregnancy is the same as OCPs. Because the delivery system is transdermal, the doses of estrogen and progestin cannot be compared directly with the doses in OCPs [60]. For example, estrogen in OCPs must undergo first pass metabolism in the liver, whereas transdermally absorbed estrogen goes directly into the circulation, so a lower dose is needed to achieve similar blood levels.

Efficacy

Zieman and colleagues evaluated the contraceptive efficacy and cycle control in 3319 women (aged 18 to 45 years) by pooling data from three multi-center, open-label contraceptive trials. From these pooled results, the overall annual probability of pregnancy (method failure plus user failure) in study participants who received the contraceptive patch was 0.88, 95% CI (0.44–1.33) [61]. Audet and colleagues published the first clinical trial of transdermal contraception. The study was a randomized, active control, multi-center clinical trial comparing the contraceptive patch with a triphasic OCP (levonorgestrel 50 μg and ethinyl estradiol 30 μg days 1 to 6, levonorgestrel 75 μg and ethinyl estradiol 40 μg days 7 to 11, levonorgestrel 125 μg and ethinyl estradiol 30 μg days 12 to 21 and placebo for days 22 to 28). It was conducted in 39 centers and enrolled 1400 participants, aged 18 to 45 years. This study found overall and method-failure Pearl Indexes were slightly lower with the transdermal patch (1.24 and 0.99, respectively) as compared with Triphasil (2.18 and 1.25, respectively), but this difference was not significant ($P = .57$) [57].

Zieman and colleagues found the transdermal patch to be less effective in a subgroup of women with a baseline body weight of at least 90 kg (at least 198 lbs). Among women who weighed less than 90 kg, the occurrence of pregnancy was infrequent, with a life-table estimate and Pearl index of 0.5% and 0.60, respectively [61]. The association between higher body weight (at least 90 kg) and increased number of contraceptive failures, however, may not be unique to transdermal hormonal contraception. Many oral contraceptive studies have excluded women who were 20% over ideal body weight; therefore the efficacy of OCPs has not been studied adequately in this subgroup of women.

Compliance and adverse events

Audet and colleagues showed that compliance with the dosing schedule of the patch was significantly better than that of OCPs. The percentage of patch cycles that demonstrated perfect compliance was 88.7% (4558 perfect patch cycles/5141 total patch cycles) as compared with 79.2% perfect compliance with OCPs (3276/4134) $P < .001$ [57].

The most frequent reported adverse effects from the patch have been documented by several studies [57,61]. Studies on adult women have found most adverse events are similar between the transdermal patch and OCP users except that patch users had a higher incidence of application site reactions, breast symptoms, defined as breast discomfort, breast pain, and breast engorgement ($P < .001$), and dysmenorrhea ($P = .04$) [61]. Most breast symptoms appear to resolve after approximately 3 months of use [57,61].

Application site reactions were found to be usually mild or moderate in severity but were a common reason cited for discontinuation of the transdermal patch [57]. Rubenstein and colleagues found 61% of adolescent patch users agreed or strongly agreed that the patch was itchy, and 13% agreed or strongly agreed that the patch gave them a rash [59].

Other adverse events reported in studies of adult women include headache (22%), nausea (17% to 20%), abdominal pain (8%), and breakthrough bleeding and spotting between menstrual cycles (18% to 10%, decreasing rates from cycle 1 to cycle 13) [57,61,62]. Adolescent patch users also reported adverse effects of increased headaches (17%), breast tenderness (31%), and spotting (10%) [59].

Contraindications

Although the transdermal patch differs from OCPs in the pharmacokinetics of estrogen and progestin delivery, the hormones in the patch are similar to those in the pill and carry the same risks and consequently have the same contraindications. Having a latex allergy does not prohibit use of the patch, as the patch is made from polyester not latex. A severe skin reaction, however, would be a reason for discontinuation.

Advantages

OrthoEvra may be a good alternative form of hormonal contraception for adolescents who have difficulty with perfect compliance with OCPs. Most OCP failures are associated with difficulty adhering to a once-a-day dosing regimen. It also has been shown that approximately 64% of adolescents discontinue OCP use within the first year [63]. More importantly, 25% of adolescents who stop the pill will be pregnant within the first year of discontinuation [63]. The patch may be a more convenient form of contraception that is easier to use because of its once-a-week dosing regimen. Although the noncontraceptive benefits of the transdermal patch have not been studied in adolescents, one can assume based on the pharmacology of the patch that these would be similar to those seen in OCPs.

Disadvantages

Although the transdermal patch appears to be as effective as OCPs, and equally tolerable, many adolescents may have difficulty with this method of contraception. Rubenstein and colleagues found that up to one third of adolescent transdermal patch users had partial or complete detachment, a higher rate than found in adult studies. These authors suggest that teens tend to be more physically active than adult users and may have higher rates of detachment based on increased physical activity and presumed body temperature and humidity changes. Nonetheless, it may serve as a barrier to use if adolescents continually are confronted with detachment and reapplication problems. In addition, the current transdermal patch is beige and does not match the skin color of nonwhite ethnic groups. Lastly, the location of the application sites may be a barrier to confidentiality. To avoid exposure of the transdermal patch, teens are limited to use sites on the buttocks and lower abdomen.

Vaginal ring combined hormonal system

The FDA approved the first vaginal ring, marketed under the name NuvaRing, in 2001. It is made of a flexible, soft, transparent ethylene vinyl acetate co-polymer. The outer diameter is 5.4 cm, with a cross-sectional diameter of 0.4 cm. This delivery system releases 120 µg of etonogestrel (ENG), a biologically active metabolite of desogestrel, and 15 µg of EE per day at a constant rate during 3 consecutive weeks. The hormones are absorbed through the vaginal mucosa directly into the circulation. As for the transdermal delivery system, the doses of hormones in the vaginal ring cannot be compared directly with the doses in OCPs that need to be higher to counteract first-pass metabolism in the liver. Each ring is inserted and removed by the user and is intended for one cycle of 3 consecutive weeks. The user removes the ring after three weeks, which allows her to have a menstrual period. According to the manufacturer, the vaginal ring can be removed for up to 3 hours during coitus if it is bothersome to the partners without requiring the use of a back -up method, but then must be reinserted by the user.

Efficacy

Trussel found vaginal ring pregnancy rates of 8% and 0.3% per woman per year for typical and perfect use, respectively [31]. The active components of the vaginal ring are based on the well-known pharmacology of estrogen and progestin and therefore work similarly to OCPs.

Roumen and colleagues published the first large-scale study evaluating the efficacy, tolerability, and acceptability of a contraceptive vaginal ring. Roumen evaluated over 800 women, aged 18 to 40 years, who used the vaginal ring over the course of 1 year. When evaluating efficacy in this study, the vaginal ring had a Pearl Index of 0.65 (95% CI 0.24 to 1.41) [64].

Compliance and adverse events

Compliance with the use of the NuvaRing was found to be 91% over a 1-year time period [64]. Spotting and breakthrough bleeding were found in 2.6% to 6.4% of the cycles [64]. Most subjects had a withdrawal bleed with a mean duration of 4.7 to 5.3 days [64]. In addition, the vaginal ring appeared to have minimal effects on lipids, with no adverse effects on blood pressure, weight, or unfavorable effects on the vagina or cervix [64]. The most frequently reported adverse reactions were vaginitis (14%), headache (12%), and leukorrhea (6%) [64]. Other adverse effects reported included nausea (5%) and vaginal discomfort (4%) [64]. The most frequently reported reason for discontinuation was device-related events (4%), including foreign body sensation, coital problems, and device expulsion [64].

Contraindications

Although the vaginal ring differs from OCPs in terms of pharmacokinetics of estrogen and progestin delivery, the hormones of the ring are similar to those of the pill and carry the same risks and consequently have the same contraindications.

Advantages

Adolescents may enjoy a reversible combined hormonal method that has an excellent safety profile, high efficacy rates, and is easy to use. The vaginal ring may fit all of these criteria. Additionally, the vaginal ring may offer adolescents the convenience once monthly dosing, as compared with the daily and weekly dosing regimens of OCPs and the transdermal patch. Similar to the transdermal patch, many of the noncontraceptive benefits offered by OCPs have not been studied in the vaginal ring but are likely to be similar.

Disadvantages

Many adolescents may feel uncomfortable with a contraception method that requires inserting a device into their vaginas. Although this was not an issue in studies of adult women, at this time there are no known studies evaluating this potential problem in adolescents. Additionally, studies in adult women have shown that common adverse effects with the vaginal ring are vaginitis (14%) and leukorrhea (6%) [64]. These symptoms may be confusing to an adolescent user who may assume she has an STI or confuse the symptoms of an STI with the effects of the ring. This may lead to an increase in worry and concern in the adolescent and ultimately lead to dissatisfaction with the method.

It also has been found that approximately 13% of women and 26% of men reported feeling the vaginal ring during intercourse, and 4% of ring users discontinued use because of device-related issues [64]. It is possible that these types of effects may cause even higher rates of discontinuation in adolescents, and this an area that warrants further study.

Injectable combined hormonal system

The injectable combined estrogen/progestin contraceptive, marketed by the name Lunelle, was approved by the FDA in 2000 but was removed from the US market by the manufacturer in 2003.

Summary

Combined estrogen and progestin contraceptives containing less than 50 μg of ethinyl estradiol are highly effective, reversible, and have a favorable risk/ benefit profile for young women. The OCP has gone through a 40-year pharmacological evolution with manipulation of the doses and chemical structure of both hormones, resulting in a choice of pills today that are safe and can be tolerated by almost any adolescent. In the past 5 years, new transdermal and transvaginal delivery systems for combined hormonal contraceptives have been marketed allowing once-a-week and once-a-month dosing, respectively that improve adherence in adult women. Experience with use of the new delivery systems in adolescents is limited, however.

It has been established that adverse events are likely to cause discontinuation, especially in adolescents. Therefore, education and counseling should be done at initiation and during the first months of method selection. Contraceptive counseling should include a discussion on how a method works, the potential adverse effects, dispelling myths, exploring barriers to use, and assurance of health care provider support.

References

[1] Santelli J, Abma J, Ventura S, et al. Can changes in sexual behaviors explain the decline in teen pregnancy rates in the 1990s? J Adolesc Health 2004;35:80–90.

[2] Ventura SJ, Abma JC, Mosher WD, et al. Estimated pregnancy rates for the United States, 1990–2000: an update. Natl Vital Stat Rep 2004;52(23):1–9.

[3] Alan Guttmacher Institute. Sex and American's teenagers. New York: The Alan Guttmacher Institute; 1994.

[4] Clark L. Will the pill make me sterile? Addressing reproductive health concerns and strategies to improve adherence to hormonal contraceptive regimens in adolescent girls. J Pediatr Adolesc Gynecol 2001;14(4):153–62.

[5] The Practice Committee of the American Society for Reproductive Medicine, American Society for Reproductive Medicine, Birmingham, Alabama. Hormonal contraception: recent advances and controversies. Fertil Steril 2004;82:520–6.

[6] Brill SR, Rosenfeld WD. Contraception. Med Clin North Am 2000;84(4):907–24.

[7] Poindexter A. The emerging use of the 20 μg oral contraceptive. Fertil Steril 2001;75(3):457–65.

[8] Meade TW, Greenberg G, Thompson SG. Progestogens and cardiovascular reactions associated with oral contraceptives and a comparison of the safety of 50 and 30 μg oestrogen preparations. BMJ 1980;280:1157–61.

[9] Lidegaard O. Oral Contraception and risk of a cerebral thromboembolic attack: results of a case control study. BMJ 1993;306:956–63.

[10] WHO Collaborative Study of Cardiovascular and Steroid Hormone Contraception. Ischemic stroke and combined oral contraceptives: results of an international, multi-center, case-control study. Lancet 1996;348:498–505.

[11] Vessey MP. Epidemiologic studies of oral contraception. Int J Fertil 1989;34:64–70.

[12] World Health Organization. Cardiovascular disease and steroid hormone contraception: report of a WHO Scientific Group. WHO Technical Report Series, No. 877. Geneva (Switzerland): World Health Organization; 1998.

[13] Dunn N, Thorogood M, Faragher B, et al. Oral contraceptives and myocardial infarction: results of the MICA case-control study. BMJ 1999;318:1579–83.

[14] Schwingl PJ, Ory HW, Visness CM. Estimates of the risk of cardiovascular death attributable to low-dose oral contraceptives in the United States. Am J Obstet Gynecol 1999;180:241–9.

[15] Rosenberg MJ, Meyers A, Roy V. Efficacy, cycle control, and side effects of low- and lower dose oral contraceptives: a randomized trial of 20 μg and 35 μg estrogen preparations. Contraception 2000;60:321–9.

[16] Abma JC, Chandra A, Mosher WD, et al. Fertility. Family planning, and women's health: new data from the 1995 National Survey of Family Growth. Vital Health Stat 1997;23(19):1–11.

[17] Hatcher RA, Trussell J, Stewart F, et al. The menstrual cycle. In: Kowal D, editor. Contraception technology. 17th revised edition. New York: Ardent Media Inc.; 1998. p. 71–6.

[18] Association of Reproductive Health Professionals. Administration of hormonal contraceptive drugs. A quick reference guide for clinicians. Available at: www.arhp.org/guide/. Accessed November 1, 2004.

[19] Rosenberg MJ, Waugh MS. Oral contraceptive discontinuation: a prospective evaluation of frequency and reasons. Am J Obstet Gynecol 1998;179:577–82.

[20] Rosenberg MJ, Long SC. Oral contraceptives and cycle control: a critical review of the literature. Adv Contracept 1992;8(Suppl 1):35–45.

[21] Brill K, Then A, Beisiegel U, et al. Investigation of the influence of two low-dose monophasic oral contraceptives containing 20 μg ethinylestradiol/75 μg gestodene and 30 μg ethinylestradiol/75 μg gestodene on lipid metabolism in an open randomized trial. Contraception 1996;54:291–7.

[22] Akerlund M. Clinical experience of a combined oral contraceptive with very low dose ethinyl estradiol. Acta Obstet Gynecol Scand 1997;164:63–5.

[23] Bannemerschult R, Hanker JP, Wunsch C, et al. A multi-center, uncontrolled clinical investigation of the contraceptive efficacy, cycle control, and safety of a new low dose oral contraceptive containing 20 μg ethinyl estradiol and 100 μg levonorgestrel over six treatment cycles. Contraception 1997;56:285–90.

[24] Archer DF, Maheux R, DelConte A, et al, North American Levonorgestrel Study Group (NALSG). A new low-dose monophasic combination oral contraceptive (Alesse) with 100 μg levonorgestrel and 20 μg ethinyl estradiol. Contraception 1997;55:139–44.

[25] Archer DF, Maheux R, DelConte A, O'Brien FB, North American Levonorgestrel Study Group (NALSG). Efficacy and safety of a low-dose monophasic combination oral contraceptive containing 100 μg levonorgestrel and 20 μg ethinyl estradiol (Alesse). Am J Obstet Gynecol 1999; 181:S39–44.

[26] Hammond GL, Rabe T, Wagner JD. Preclinical profiles of progestins used in formulations of oral contraceptives and hormone replacement therapy. Am J Obstet Gynecol 2001;185: S24–31.

[27] Carr BR. Uniqueness of oral contraceptive progestins. Contraception 1998;58(Suppl 3):23–7.

[28] Phillips A, Demarest K, Hahn DW, et al. Progestional and androgenic receptor binding affinities and in vivo activities of norgestimate and other progestins. Contraception 1990;41:399–410.

[29] Upmalis D, Phillips A. Receptor binding and in vivo activities of the new progestins. J Soc Obstet Gynaecol Canada 1991;13:35–9.

[30] Rabe T, Kowald A, Ortmann J, et al. Inhibition of skin 5-alpha reductase by oral contraceptive progestins in vitro. Gynecol Endocrinol 2000;14:223–30.

[31] Trussell J. Contraceptive failure in the United States. Contraception 2004;70:89–96.

[32] Rosenberg MJ, Waugh MS, Meehan TE. Use and misuse of oral contraceptives: risk indicators for poor pill taking and discontinuation. Contraception 1995;51:283–8.

[33] Emans SJ, Grace E, Woods ER, et al. Adolescents' compliance with the use of oral contraceptives. JAMA 1987;257:3377–81.

[34] Meyers AB, Rhodes JE. Oral contraceptive use among African American adolescents: individual and community influences. Am J Community Psychol 1995:99–115.

[35] Collaborative Group on Hormonal Factors in Breast Cancer. Breast cancer and hormonal contraceptives: collaborative reanalysis of individual data on 53, 297 women with breast cancer

and 100, 239 women without breast cancer form 54 epidemiological studies. Lancet 1996; 347:1713–27.

[36] Petitti DB, Sidney S, Bernstein A, et al. Stroke in users of low-dose oral contraceptives. N Engl J Med 1996;335:8–15.

[37] Schwartz SM, Petitti DB, Siscovick DS, et al. Stroke and the use of low-dose oral contraceptives in young women: a pooled analysis of 2 US studies. Stroke 1998;29:2277–84.

[38] Sidney S, Siscovick DS, Petitti DB, et al. Myocardial infarction and the use of low-dose oral contraceptives: a pooled analysis of 2 US studies. Circulation 1998;98:1058–63.

[39] Wilks JF. Hormonal birth control and pregnancy: a comparative analysis of thromboembolic risk. Ann Pharmacother 2003;37:912–6.

[40] Chapdelaine A, Desmarais JL, Derman R. Clinical evidence of the minimal androgenic activity of norgestimate. Int J Fertil 1989;34:347–52.

[41] Lobo RA, Skinner JB, Lippman JS, et al. Plasma lipids and desogestrel and ethinyl estradiol: a meta-analysis. Fertil Steril 1996;65:1100–9.

[42] LaRosa JC. Effects of oral contraceptives on circulating lipids and lipoproteins; maximizing benefit, minimizing risk. Int J Fertil 1989;34:71–84.

[43] Parsey KS, Pong A. An open-label, multi-center study to evaluate Yasmin, a low-dose combination oral contraceptive containind drospirenone, a new progestin. Contraception 2000;61: 105–11.

[44] World Health Organization. Improving access to quality care in family planning: medical eligibility for contraceptive use. 2nd edition. Geneva (Switzerland): World Health Organization; 2000.

[45] Derman R. Oral contraceptives, assessment of benefits. J Reprod Med 1986;31(9):879–86.

[46] Dayal M, Barnhart K. Noncontraceptive benefits and therapeutic uses of the oral contraceptive pill. Seminars in Reproductive Medicine 2001;19(4):295–303.

[47] Peterson LS, Oakley D, Potter LS, et al. Womens' efforts to prevent pregnancy: consistency of oral contraceptive use. Fam Plann Perspect 1998;30:19.

[48] Hillard PJ. Oral contraception noncompliance: the extent of the problem. Adv Contracept 1992; 8:13–20.

[49] Serfaty D. Medical aspects of oral contraceptive discontinuation. Adv Contracept 1992;8: 21–33.

[50] Muhn P, Krattenmacher R, Beier S, et al. Drospirenone: a novel progestogen with anti-mineralocorticoid and antiandrogenic activity. Pharmacological characterization in animal models. Contraception 1995;51:99–110.

[51] Advisory Board for the New Progestins, Speroff L, DeCherney A. Evaluation of a new generation of oral contraceptives. Obstet Gynecol 1993;81:1034–47.

[52] Schwetz B. New Oral Contraceptive. JAMA 2001;285(5):527.

[53] Anderson FD, Hait H, and the Seasonale-301 Study Group. A multi-center, randomized study of an extended cycle oral contraceptive. Contraception 2003;68:89–96.

[54] Sulak PJ, Cressman BE, Waldorp E, et al. Extending the duration of active oral contraceptive pills to manage hormone withdrawal symptoms. Obstet Gynecol 1997;89:179–83.

[55] Chacko MR, Kozinetz CA, Smith PB. Assessment of oral contraceptive pill continuation in young women. J Pediatr Adolesc Gynecol 1999;12:143–8.

[56] Fu H, Darroch JE, Haas T, et al. Contraceptive failure rates: new estimates from the 1995 National Survey of Family Growth. Fam Plann Perspect 1999;31:56–63.

[57] Audet MC, Moreau M, Koltun W, et al. Evaluation of contraceptive efficacy and cycle control of a transdermal contraceptive patch vs. an oral contraceptive. JAMA 2001;285(18):2347–54.

[58] Skee D, Abrams LS, Natarajan J, Anderson GD, Wong F. Pharmacokinetics of a contraceptive patch at 4 application sites. Clin Pharmacol Ther 2000;67:159.

[59] Rubinstein ML, Halpern-Felsher BL, Irwin CE. An evaluation of the use of the transdermal contraceptive patch in adolescents. J Adolesc Health 2004;34:395–401.

[60] Abrms L, Skee D, Talluri K, et al. Bioavailability of 17-deacetylnorgestimate (17D-NGM) and ethinyl estradiol (EE) from a contraceptive patch. FASEB J 2000;14:A1479.

[61] Zieman M, Guillebaud J, Weisberg E, et al. Contraceptive efficacy and cycle control with the

Ortho Evra/Evra transdermal system: the analysis of pooled data. Fertil Steril 2002;77(Suppl 2): S13–8.

[62] Sibai BM, Odlind V, Meador ML, et al. A comparative and pooled analysis of the safety and tolerability of the contraceptive patch (Ortho Evra/Evra). Fertil Steril 2002;77(Suppl 2):S19–26.

[63] Berenson AB, Wiemann CM, Rickert VI, et al. Contraceptive outcomes among adolescents prescribed Norplant implants versus oral contraceptives after one year of use. Am J Obstet Gynecol 1997;176:586–92.

[64] Roumen FJME, Apter D, Mulders TMT, et al. Efficacy, tolerability and acceptability of a novel contraceptive vaginal ring releasing etonogestrel and ethinyl oestradiol. Hum Reprod 2001; 16(3):469–75.

ELSEVIER
SAUNDERS

ADOLESCENT
MEDICINE
CLINICS

Adolesc Med 16 (2005) 539–551

Hormonal Contraception: Noncontraceptive Benefits and Medical Contraindications

Kristin M. Rager, MD, MPH, Hatim A. Omar, MD*

*Section of Adolescent Medicine, University of Kentucky College of Medicine, J 422 Kentucky Clinic,
Lexington, KY 40536-0284, USA*

Hormonal contraception is used primarily for the benefit of protection from pregnancy. Recent studies have demonstrated many noncontraceptive benefits also. Most young women, however, are unaware of these benefits [1]. In counseling patients about hormonal contraception, it is essential to discuss the health benefits in addition to adverse effects and risks, as increased knowledge of the noncontraceptive benefits of birth control methods can increase compliance and continuation of use, with the ultimate goal of decreasing unplanned pregnancy.

Noncontraceptive benefits of oral contraceptive pills (combined)

Decreased ovarian cancers

Use of combination oral contraceptive pills (COCPs) repeatedly has been demonstrated to decrease the risk of developing ovarian cancer. Women with a history of any COCP use have 40% to 50% reduced rates of ovarian cancer [2–4]. A meta-analysis of 20 prior studies noted a protective effect in 18 studies, with a summary relative risk of 0.64 (95% confidence interval [CI] = 0.57 to 0.73) [5]. This protective effect has been shown to increase with duration of COCP use [2]. The mechanism of protection is thought to be related to suppression of ovulation, as in multi-parous women and those with prolonged breastfeeding [6]. In addition, a 60% reduction in risk (95% CI = 0.2 to 0.7) was noted in those women positive for breast cancer genetic mutations who had used COCP in the past [3].

---

* Corresponding author.
E-mail address: haomar2@uky.edu (H.A. Omar).

Decreased endometrial cancer

Endometrial cancer risk also has been demonstrated to decrease with use of COCP. Women who have used COCPs have a reduction in endometrial cancer risk of up to 90% [2,7,8]. There is evidence that this protective effect increases with duration of COCP use [2]. It is hypothesized that combined COCP use reduces endometrial cancer risk through the action of progestins that reduce endometrial mitotic rate [9].

Decreased colorectal cancer

Data on protection from colorectal cancer are inconsistent. A 1998 meta-analysis found that three of four cohort studies and 5 of 11 case-control studies demonstrated a reduced risk of colorectal cancer in women who had ever used COCPs versus women who had never used COCPs [10]. In a more recent meta-analysis, the pooled estimate from all studies combined was 0.82 (95% CI: 0.74 to 0.92). Duration of use was not associated with a decrease in risk, but there was some indication that the apparent protection was stronger for women who had used COCPs more recently (relative risk = 0.46; 95% CI: 0.30 to 0.71) [11]. Cell proliferation in the colon is inhibited by estrogen through receptors in the colonic epithelium [12].

Decreased ovarian cysts

Studies regarding ovarian cysts are also conflicting. Functional cysts of the ovary occurred much less commonly in women who had taken COCPs in the 6 months prior (35 μg estrogen content) than in those who had taken them in the past or never before. Corpus luteum cysts decreased by 78% (95% CI = 47% to 93%), and follicular cysts by 49% (95% CI = 20% to 70%). The authors estimated that about 28 (95% CI = 16 to 35) operations for functional ovarian cysts could be avoided among every 100,000 women taking COCPs each year [13]. A dose gradient seems to exist for the suppression of functional cysts. A 76% reduction was seen in those given 50 μg ethinyl estradiol monophasic pills or higher, and a 48% reduction was seen in those given less than 50 μg ethinyl estradiol monophasics [14]. Three recent studies, however, found no effect on functional cysts with low-dose (less than 35 μg ethinyl estradiol) combination pills [15–17].

Decreased acne

Combination OCPs have demonstrated statistically significant improvements in acne: decreased inflammatory lesions by up to 62% and decreased total lesions by up to 53% [18,19]. This is thought to be secondary to decreased free testosterone because of increased sex hormone binding globulin (SHBG) [18]. Many providers consider COCPs an acceptable second-line treatment for acne, and COCPs recently gained US Food and Drug Administration (FDA) approval for this indication.

Decreased benign breast disease

Risk of benign breast disease (BBD) was found to decrease significantly with a longer use of COCPs before the first full-term pregnancy, but there was no association after. These results were independent of estrogen content [20]. There was an inverse association between the use of COCPs and risk of all types of BBD combined, and risk progressively decreased with increasing duration of use. COCP use for more than 7 years yielded a decreased risk of 36% (95% CI = 0.68 to 3.01) [21].

Decreased salpingitis

Risk for salpingitis may be reduced by up to 80% in women currently using combined oral contraceptives [22,23]. Among current users who had been using COCPs for greater than 12 months, the risk of pelvic inflammatory disease (PID) was decreased by half (95% CI = 0.4 to 0.6). Past use did not exert a protective effect [24]. Among women with chlamydia, risk of PID was 80% less than in those not using COCP; however, no significant association was seen in those with gonorrhea [23]. It is estimated that 50,000 cases of PID and 12,500 hospitalizations are avoided each year by use of COCPs [24], with up to a 60% decreased risk of hospitalization for those on COCPs who do develop PID [23–26].

Decreased ectopic pregnancy

Meta-analysis of the association between contraceptive method and risk of ectopic pregnancies found that COCPs protect against ectopic pregnancies, with approximately 90% reduction in risk [22,27]. If women on COCPs do become pregnant, they are much less likely to develop an ectopic pregnancy.

Decreased dysmenorrhea and menorrhagia

As a primary mechanism of action, combined COCPs prevent pregnancy by inhibiting ovulation. This is also the theorized mechanism for the associated decreases in menstrual-associated adverse effects, such as dysmenorrhea and menorrhagia. Current COCP use decreases prevalence and severity of dysmenorrhea [28,29]. By inhibiting ovulation, COCPs decrease uterine activity and responsiveness to agonists such as $PGF2\alpha$ [30]. Menstrual blood loss and duration of flow also is decreased significantly on COCPs [29–32]. Blood loss with menstruation is decreased in all women on COCPs by as much as 40% after 3 months of use. The most notable decrease occurs during the first 2 days of menstruation [29]. In short, COCP are quite effective in managing dysmenorrhea and menorrhagia and are recommended as first-line treatment for dysmenorrhea associated with endometriosis [33].

Improved symptoms in polycystic ovary syndrome

Combined OCPs effectively treat the symptoms of polycystic ovary syndrome (PCOS) such as acne, hirsutism, and dysfunctional uterine bleeding. Use of COCPs for 3 months improved bleeding patterns and baseline physical functioning, such as self-care, walking, lifting, and exercising, in greater than 80% of PCOS subjects with dysfunctional uterine bleeding [34,35].

Decreased iron deficiency anemia

Women currently using COCPs had menstrual bleeding of significantly shorter duration (and therefore higher ferritin levels) than those using other methods [36,37]. The increased iron stores seen in women on COCPs are related to the decreased menstrual blood loss and duration of menses.

Decreased osteoporosis

Women on COCPs either maintained or increased bone mineral density, whereas controls lost bone mineral density [38,39]. Increased effects were seen with increased exposure, especially in the first 5 years [40]. Women who had ever used any COCP had 25% (95% CI 0.59 to 0.96) decreased risk, and women who had ever used high-dose COCPs had a 44% (95% CI = 0.42 to 0.75) decreased risk for hip fractures when compared with those who had never used COCPs [41].

Decreased fibroids

There is a significantly reduced risk of fibroids among past and current COCP users, and this risk decreases with longer use [42]. Current users demonstrated a 70% reduction in fibroids (95% CI = 0.2 to 0.6), and past users who used COCP for 7 or more years had a 50% reduction in fibroids (95% CI = 0.3 to 0.9) [43].

Other combined delivery systems

Although there have been no independent studies, it is expected that the noncontraceptive benefits of COCPs will be found in other combined methods, such as the once-a-week birth control patch (and the contraceptive ring.

Noncontraceptive benefits of progestin-only methods

Scanty or no menses

Depot medroxyprogesterone acetate (DMPA) often has adverse effects of irregular bleeding. Forty six percent of women reported amenorrhea after 3 months of DMPA, 53% after 6 months, and 58.5% after 9 months [44]. A comparable study found 60% amenorrhea at days 121 to 240 after first injection and 73% during days 241 to 360 [45]. This often is viewed as a benefit, as 72% of women 13.5 to 21 years old reported being very happy with the amenorrhea from using DMPA [46]. In addition, a suggested benefit of the amenorrhea from DMPA is for menstrual control in mentally handicapped women with menstrual hygiene problems [47].

Decreased endometrial cancer

Depot medroxyprogesterone acetate has been shown to decrease the risk of endometrial cancer for all users [48] and by almost 80% in women who used DMPA for more than 1 year before diagnosis [49].

Decreased pelvic inflammatory disease

Current DMPA use has be shown to decrease risk of developing PID. This is thought to be caused by thickening of cervical mucous and therefore decreased movement of pathogens into the upper genital tract [50,51].

Decreased ectopic pregnancy

Women who report a history of DMPA use have a decreased risk of ectopic pregnancies versus women who report using no contraception [52].

Decreased seizure frequency

Use of DMPA in patients with seizure disorders is suggested to decrease frequency of seizures [53,54]. In addition, DMPA does not interfere with the metabolism of any current antiseizure medications.

Does not interfere with breastfeeding

Depot medroxyprogesterone acetate is a safe and preferred method of hormonal contraception for the breastfeeding woman. Neither DMPA nor progestin-only pills decrease duration of lactation or lessen infant weight gain when given postpartum [55–57].

Specific contraindications to oral contraceptive pills (combined)

In 2004, the World Health Organization (WHO) published its third edition of the Medical Eligibility Criteria for Contraceptive Use. Medical conditions are assigned to a category of eligibility for patient use. Categories 3 (a condition where the theoretical or proven risks usually outweigh the advantages of using the method) and 4 (a condition that represents an unacceptable health risk if the contraceptive method is used) indicate that use of the contraceptive method is not recommended. Conditions assigned to Category 3 for low-dose combined oral contraceptives (no more than 35 μg ethinyl estradiol), the patch, and the ring are listed in Box 1 [58]. Conditions assigned to Category 4 for low-dose combined

---

Box 1. Medical conditions where the theoretical or proven risks usually outweigh the advantages of using low-dose combined oral contraceptives (COC), the patch (P) or the ring (R)

Primarily breastfeeding ≥ 6 weeks to < 6 months postpartum
Nonbreastfeeding < 6 weeks postpartum (COC only)
Nonbreastfeeding < 21 days postpartum (P/R only)
Age ≥ 35 years, smoking < 15 cigarettes/d
Multiple risk factors for arterial cardiovascular disease (such as older age, smoking, diabetes, or hypertension)
History of hypertension where blood pressure cannot be evaluated
Adequately controlled hypertension, where blood pressure can be evaluated
Elevated blood pressure levels (systolic 140–159 or diastolic 90–99)
Known hyperlipidemias[a]
Migraine without aura, age < 35 years (to continue oc)
Migraine without aura, age ≥ 35 years (to initiate oc)
Past breast cancer with no evidence of current disease for 5 years
Diabetes with nephropathy/neuropathy/retinopathy[b]
Diabetes with other vascular disease or for > 20 years duration*
Medically treated symptomatic gall bladder disease
Current symptomatic gall bladder disease
Past oc-related cholestasis
Mild (compensated) cirrhosis
Current use of rifampin
Current use of anticonvulsants, such as phenytoin, carbamazepine, barbiturates, primidone, topiramate, or oxcarbazepine

[a] Category 2/3.
[b] Category 3/4.

oral contraceptives, the patch, and the ring, are listed in Box 2 [58]. These recommendations are to be used as a guideline in combination with clinical judgment on a patient-by-patient basis. Specific issues, such as venous thromboembolism, cardiovascular disease, and headache warrant further discussion.

Venous thromboembolism

Older studies of high-dose (50 μg of ethinyl estradiol or mestranol) COCPs found a significant association between COCP use and venous thromboembolism (VTE). More recently, high-dose COCPs have been found to increase clotting factors VII, VIII, X, XII, protein C, and fibrinogen, and to decrease antithrombin III and protein S [58]. A 1997 meta-analysis of 22 studies found the pooled risk of idiopathic VTE among users of low-dose COCP to be 2.4 to 4.8 times greater than that among nonusers [59]. The highest increase in risk has been suggested to be in the first year of use [60]. Other studies, however, have con-

---

Box 2. Medical conditions where using low-dose combined oral contraceptives (COC), the patch (P), or the ring (R) represents an unacceptable health risk

Breastfeeding < 6 weeks postpartum
Age ≥ 35 years, smoking ≥ 15 cigarettes/d
Multiple risk factors for arterial cardiovascular disease*
Elevated blood pressure levels (systolic > 160 or diastolic > 100)
Hypertension with vascular disease
History of DVT/PE
Current DVT/PE
Major surgery with prolonged immobilization
Known thrombogenic mutations (eg, factor V Leiden, prothrombin mutation, protein C or S, or antithrombin deficiency)
Current and history of ischaemic heart disease
History of cerebrovascular accident
Complicated valvular heart disease
Migraine without aura, age ≥ 35 years (to continue)
Migraine with aura, any age
Current breast cancer
Diabetes with nephropathy/neuropathy/retinopathy*
Diabetes with other vascular disease or for > 20 years duration*
Active viral hepatitis
Severe (decompensated) cirrhosis
Liver tumors (benign or malignant)

* Category 3/4.

cluded that low-dose COCPs have no significant clinical impact on the coagulation system [61,62]. One hypothesis is that a significant number of those cases where a patient on low-dose COCP has developed VTE may be attributed to inherited clotting disorders. Heterozygotes for factor V Leiden mutation (the most common inherited clotting disorder) have an eight-fold increased risk of VTE, and homozygotes have an 80-fold increased risk above the general population. This risk appears to be increased by 30-fold in those on COCPs [63]. Prothrombin mutation is the second most common inherited clotting disorder, and COCP use has been reported to markedly increase the risk of VTE in these patients also [64]. Use of COCP in patients with known heritable clotting disorders therefore is discouraged strongly.

Cardiovascular disease

The nurses' Health Study found an association between past use of COCP and increased risk of cardiovascular disease (CVD) [65]. Other studies have not supported this finding in women on COCPs who do not smoke [66,67]. This risk is elevated significantly in women who use COCPs and smoke cigarettes. Women who smoke heavily and use even very low-dose COCPs (less than 20 µg ethinyl estradiol) have an increased risk of myocardial infarction [66]. Estrogen, however, has been found to raise plasma concentrations of high-density lipoprotein cholesterol while lowering concentrations of low-density lipoprotein cholesterol and improving endothelial vascular function [68].

Stroke and transient ischemic attacks

Among 626 women with a history of cerebral thrombotic event, when women who had ever used COCPs were compared with nonusers, those taking a high-dose COCP had 4.5 times increased risk, while those on low-dose COCPs had a 1.7 times increased risk [69].

Headaches

A 1995 study of women and migraines found that 30% of the women with migraines were currently using COCPs [70]. Migraines without aura generally improve on COCPs; however, in women on COCPs, migraine with aura may worsen, or attacks with aura may occur for the first time [71]. In addition, women with a history of migraine with aura and who take COCPs have a 3.2 to 6.8 times increased risk of stroke [72–74]. Those who have migraines with aura, who take COCPs and smoke cigarettes, have a 34.4 times increased risk of stroke [74]. It therefore is advised that women who have a history of migraines with aura do not use COCPs, especially if they smoke.

Specific contraindications to progestin only methods

Medical conditions assigned by the WHO to Categories 3 and 4 for DMPA/progestin only pills (POP) are listed in Box 3 [75]. Again, these are to be used as guidelines in concert with clinical judgment.

Venous thromboembolism and cardiovascular disease

Although it is suggested otherwise in the WHO guidelines, progestin only contraceptives, unlike COCPs, have been shown to have no effect on the clotting

---

Box 3. Medical conditions where the theoretical or proven risks usually outweigh the advantages of using progestin-only pills (POP) or depot medroxyprogesterone acetate/norethisterone enanthate (D/NE)

Breastfeeding <6 weeks postpartum
Multiple risk factors for cardiovascular disease[a]
Elevated blood pressure (systolic >160 or diastolic >100)
Hypertension with vascular disease[b]
Current DVT/PE
Current and history of ischaemic heart disease[b]
History of cerebrovascular accident[b]
Migraine with aura at any age (to continue method)
Unexplained vaginal bleeding[a]
Past breast cancer with no evidence of current disease for 5 years
Diabetes with nephropathy/neuropathy/retinopathy[a]
Diabetes with other vascular disease or for >20 years duration[a]
Active viral hepatitis
Severe (decompensated) cirrhosis
Liver tumors (benign or malignant)
Current use of rifampin[c]
Current use of anticonvulsants, such as phenytoin, carbamazepine, barbiturates, primidone, topiramate, or oxcarbazepine[c]

Medical conditions where using progestin-only contraceptives represents an unacceptable health risk

Current breast cancer

[a] D/NE.
[b] Category 2/3.
[c] POP.

pathway [76]. In addition, the American College of Obstetrics and Gynecology states that DMPA may be used safely by women at risk for arterial or venous events [77] and bears no increased risk of stroke or transient ischemic attack [69].

Summary

Hormonal contraception has been used for decades as protection against undesired pregnancy. Many young women are unaware of the noncontraceptive benefits provided by hormonal contraception [1]. A minority, however, cite contraception as their most important reason for use [78]. Providers often do a great job of counseling patients on the contraindications to hormonal contraception, the risks associated with hormonal contraception, and the potential adverse effects. They should include the noncontraceptive benefits of hormonal contraception in the patient education repertoire, as knowledge of these benefits may be integral in promoting continued and correct use, therefore decreasing unplanned pregnancies in young women.

References

[1] Kaunitz A. Oral contraceptive health benefits: perception versus reality. Contraception 1999;59: 29S–33S.

[2] Schlesselman JJ. Net effect of oral contraceptive use on the risk of cancer in women in the United States. Obstet Gynecol 1995;85:793–801.

[3] Narod SA, Risch H, Moslehi R, et al. Oral contraceptives and the risk of hereditary ovarian cancer. Hereditary Ovarian Cancer Clinical Study Group. N Engl J Med 1998;339:424–8.

[4] Ness RB, Grisso JA, Vergona R, et al. Oral contraceptives, other methods of contraception, and risk reduction for ovarian cancer. Epidemiology 2001;12:307–12.

[5] Hankinson SE, Colditz GA, Hunter DJ, et al. A quantitative assessment of oral contraceptive use and risk of ovarian cancer. Obstet Gynecol 1992;80:708–14.

[6] Gwinn ML, Lee NC, Rhodes PH, et al. Pregnancy, breastfeeding, and oral contraceptives and the risk of epithelial ovarian cancer. J Clin Epidemiol 1990;43:559–68.

[7] Sherman M, Sturgeon S, Brinton LA, et al. Risk factors and hormone levels in patients with serous and endometrioid uterine carcinomas. Mod Pathol 1997;10:963–8.

[8] Vessey MP, Painter R. Endometrial and ovarian cancer and oral contraceptives—findings in a large cohort study. Br J Cancer 1995;71:1340–2.

[9] Key TJ, Pike MC. The dose-effect relationship between unopposed oestrogens and endometrial mitotic rate: its central role in explaining and predicting endometrial cancer risk. Br J Cancer 1988;57(2):205–12.

[10] Franceschi S, La Vecchia C. Oral contraceptives and colorectal tumors: a review of epidemiologic studies. Contraception 1998;58:335–43.

[11] Fernandez E, La Vecchia C. Oral contraceptives and colorectal cancer risk: a meta-analysis. Br J Cancer 2001;84(5):722–7.

[12] Martinez ME, Grodstein F, Giovannucci E, et al. A prospective study of reproductive factors, oral contraceptive use, and risk of colorectal cancer. Cancer Epidemiol Biomarkers Prev 1997;6:1–5.

[13] Vessey M, Metcalfe A, Wells C, et al. Ovarian neoplasms, functional ovarian cysts, and oral contraceptives. BMJ (Clin Res Ed) 1987;294(6586):1518–20.

[14] Lanes S, Birmann B, Walker AM, et al. Oral contraceptive type and functional ovarian cysts. Am J Obstet Gynecol 1992;166:956–61.

[15] Grimes DA, Godwin AJ, Rubin A, et al. Ovulation and follicular development associated with three low-dose oral contraceptives: a randomized controlled trial. Obstet Gynecol 1994;83: 29–34.

[16] Chiaffarino F, Parazzini F, La Vecchia C, et al. Oral contraceptive use and benign gynecologic conditions: a review. Contraception 1998;57:11–8.

[17] Young RL, Snabes MC, Frank ML, et al. A randomized, double-blind, placebo-controlled comparison of the impact of low-dose and triphasic oral contraceptives on follicular development. Am J Obstet Gynecol 1992;167:678–82.

[18] Lucky AW, Henderson TA, Olson WH, et al. Effectiveness of norgestimate and ethinyl estradiol in treating moderate acne vulgaris. J Am Acad Dermatol 1997;37(5):746–54.

[19] Redmond GP, Olson WH, Lippman JS, et al. Norgestimate and ethinyl estradiol in the treatment of acne vulgaris: a randomized, placebo-controlled trial. Obstet Gynecol 1997;89(4):615–22.

[20] Charreau I, Plu-Bureau G, Bachelot A, et al. Oral contraceptive use and risk of benign breast disease in a French case-control study of young women. Eur J Cancer Prev 1993;2(2):147–54.

[21] Rohan TE, Miller AB. A cohort study of oral contraceptive use and benign breast disease. Int J Cancer 1999;82(2):191–6.

[22] Petersen HB, Lee NC. The health effects of oral contraceptives: misperceptions, controversies, and continuing good news. Clin Obstet Gynecol 1989;32:339–55.

[23] Wolner-Hanssen P, Svensson L, Mardh PA, et al. Laparoscopic findings and contraceptive use in women with signs and symptoms suggestive of acute salpingitis. Obstet Gynecol 1985;66: 233–8.

[24] Rubin GL, Ory HW, Layde PM. Oral contraceptives and pelvic inflammatory disease. Am J Obstet Gynecol 1982;144:630–5.

[25] Wolner-Hanssen P, Eschenbach DA, Paavonen J, et al. Decreased risk of symptomatic chlamydial pelvic inflammatory disease associated with oral contraceptive use. JAMA 1990;263: 54–9.

[26] Panser LA, Phipps WR. Type of oral contraceptive in relation to acute, initial episodes of pelvic inflammatory disease. Contraception 1991;43:91–9.

[27] Mol BW, Ankum WM, Bossuyt PM, et al. Contraception and the risk of ectopic pregnancy: a meta-analysis. Contraception 1995;52:337–41.

[28] Milsom I, Sundell G, Andersch B. The influence of different combined oral contraceptives on the prevalence and severity of dysmenorrhea. Contraception 1990;42:497–506.

[29] Larsson G, Milsom I, Lindstedt G, et al. The influence of a low-dose combined oral contraceptive on menstrual blood loss and iron status. Contraception 1992;46:327–34.

[30] Hauksson A, Ekström P, Juchnicka E, et al. The influence of a combined oral contraceptive on uterine activity and reactivity to agonists in primary dysmenorrhea. Acta Obstet Gynecol Scand 1989;68:31–4.

[31] Fraser I, McCarron G. Randomized trial of 2 hormonal and 2 prostaglandin-inhibition agents in women with a complaint of menorrhagia. Aust NZ J Obstet Gynecol 1991;31:66–70.

[32] Iyer V, et al. Oral contraceptive pills for heavy menstrual bleeding. Cochrane Database Syst Rev 1999;3:3.

[33] Moore J, Kennedy S, Prentice A. Modern combined oral contraceptives for pain associated with endometriosis. Cochrane Database Syst Rev 2000;2:CD001019.

[34] Davis A, Godwin A, Lippman J, et al. Triphasic norgestimate-ethinyl estradiol for treating dysfunctional uterine bleeding. Obstet Gynecol 2000;96(6):913–20.

[35] Pfeifer S. Treatment of the adolescent patient with polycystic ovary syndrome. Obstet Gynecol Clin North Am 2003;30(2):337–52.

[36] Milman N. Iron status in 268 Danish women aged 18–30 years: influence of menstruation, contraceptive method, and iron supplementation. Ann Hematol 1998;77:13–9.

[37] Galan P, Yoon HC, Preziosi P, et al. Determining factors in the iron status of adult women in the SU.VI.MAX study. Supplementation en Vitamines et Mineraux Antioxydants. Eur J Clin Nutr 1998;52(6):383–8.

[38] Williams J. Noncontraceptive benefits of oral contraceptive use: an evidence based approach. Int J Fertil Womens Med 2000;45:241–7.

[39] Lindsay R, Tohme J, Kauders B. The effect of oral contraceptive use on vertebral bone mass in pre-and post-menopausal women. Contraception 1986;34:333–40.

[40] Pasco J, Kotowicz MA, Henry MJ, et al. Oral contraceptives and bone mineral density: a population-based study. Am J Obstet Gynecol 2000;182(2):265–9.

[41] Michaelsson K, Baron JA, Farahmand BY, et al. Oral contraceptive use and risk of hip fracture: a case-control study. Lancet 1999;353(9163):1481–4.

[42] Ross RK, Pike MC, Vessey MP, et al. Risk factors for uterine fibroids: reduced risk associated with oral contraceptives. BMJ 1986;293(6543):359–62.

[43] Chiaffarino F, Parazzini F, La Vecchia C, et al. Use of oral contraceptives and uterine fibroids: results from a case-control study. Br J Obstet Gynaecol 1999;106:857–60.

[44] Sangi-Haghpeykar H, Poindexter AN, Bateman L, et al. Experiences of injectable contraceptive users in an urban setting. Obstet Gynecol 1996;88:227.

[45] Mainvaring R, et al. Metabolic parameters, bleeding, and weight changes in US women using progestin-only contraceptives. J Reprod Med 1995;51:149.

[46] Smith RD, Cromer BA, Hayes JR, et al. Medroxyprogesterone acetate (Depo-Provera) use in adolescents: uterine bleeding and blood pressure patterns, patient satisfaction, and continuation rates. Adolesc Pediatr Gynecol 1995;8:24.

[47] Elkins TE, Gafford S, Muram D. A model clinic approach to the reproductive health concerns of the mentally handicapped. Obstet Gynecol 1986;68:185.

[48] Kaunitz AM. Depot medroxyprogesterone acetate contraception and the risk of breast and gynecologic cancer. J Reprod Med 1996;41(Suppl 5):419.

[49] Gray R. Reduced risk of pelvic inflammatory disease with injectable contraceptives. Lancet 1985;1:1046.

[50] Cullins V. Noncontraceptive benefits and therapeutic uses of depot medroxyprogesterone acetate. J Reprod Med 1996;41(Suppl 5):428.

[51] World Health Organization Collaborative Study of Neoplasia and Steroid Contraceptives. Depot-medroxyprogesterone acetate (DMPA) and risk of endometrial cancer. Int J Cancer 1991; 49:191.

[52] Gray RH, Pardthaisong T. In utero exposure to steroid contraceptives and survival during infancy. Am J Epidemiol 1991;134:804–11.

[53] Mattson RH, Cramer JA, Darney PD, et al. Use of oral contraceptives by women with epilepsy. JAMA 1986;256(2):238–40.

[54] Mattson RH, Rebar RW. Contraceptive methods for women with neurologic disorders. Am J Obstet Gynecol 1993;168:2027–32.

[55] Guiloff E, Ibarra-Polo A, Zañartu J, et al. Effect of contraception on lactation. Am J Obstet Gynecol 1974;118:42.

[56] Halderman L. Impact of early postpartum administration of progestin-only hormonal contraceptives compared with nonhormonal contraceptives on short-term breast-feeding patterns. Am J Obstet Gynecol 2002;186(6):1250–6.

[57] Truitt S. Combined hormonal versus nonhormonal versus progestin-only contraception in lactation. Cochrane Database Syst Rev 2003;2:CD003988.

[58] Bloemenkamp KW, Rosendaal FR, Helmerhorst FM, et al. Hemostatic effects of oral contraceptives in women who developed deep-vein thrombosis while using oral contraceptives. Thromb Haemost 1998;80:382.

[59] Douketis JD, Ginsberg JS, Holbrook A, et al. A re-evaluation of the risk for venous thromboembolism with the use of oral contraceptives and hormone replacement therapy. Arch Intern Med 1997;157(14):1522–30.

[60] Lidegaard O, Edstrom B, Kreiner S. Oral contraceptives and venous thromboembolism: a five-year national case-control study. Contraception 2002;65(3):187–96.

[61] Jespersen J, Peterson KR, Skouby SO. Effects of newer oral contraceptives on the inhibition of coagulation and fibrinolysis in relation to dosage and type of steroid. Am J Obstet Gynecol 1990;396:163.

[62] Notelovitz M, Kitchens CS, Khan FY. Changes in coagulation and anticoagulation in women taking low-dose triphasic oral contraceptives: a controlled comparative 12-month clinical trial. Am J Obstet Gynecol 1992;167:1255.

[63] Vandenbroucke JP, Koster T, Briet E, et al. Increased risk of venous thrombosis in oral – contraceptive users who are carriers of factor V Leiden mutation. Lancet 1994;344:1453.

[64] Martinelli I, Taioli E, Bucciarelli P, et al. Interaction between the G20210A mutation of the prothrombin gene and oral contraceptive use in deep vein thrombosis. Arterioscler Thromb Vasc Biol 1999;19:700.

[65] Stampfer MJ, Willett WC, Colditz GA, et al. Past use of oral contraceptives and cardiovascular disease: a meta-analysis in the context of the nurses' health study. Am J Obstet Gynecol 1990; 163:285.

[66] Basdevant A, Conard J, Pelissier C, et al. Hemostatic and metabolic effects of lowering the ethinyl-estradiol dose from 30 mcg to 20 mcg in oral contraceptives containing desogestrel. Contraception 1993;48:193–203.

[67] World Health Organization Collaborative Study of Cardiovascular Disease and Steroid Hormone Contraception. Acute myocardial infarction and combined oral contraceptives: results of an international multi-centre case-control study. Lancet 1997;349:1202–9.

[68] Mendelsohn ME, Karas RH. The protective effects of estrogen on the cardiovascular system. N Engl J Med 1999;340:1801–11.

[69] Lidegaard O. Contraceptives and cerebral thrombosis: a five-year national case-control study. Contraception 2002;65(3):197–205.

[70] Johannes CB, Linet MS, Stewart WF, et al. Relationship of headache to the phase of the menstrual cycle among young women: a daily diary study. Neurology 1995;45:1076–82.

[71] MacGregor E. Oestrogen and attacks of migraine with and without aura. Lancet Neurol 2004; 3(6):354–61.

[72] Tzourio C, Tchindrazanarivelo A, Iglesias S, et al. Case-control study of migraine and risk of ischaemic stroke in young women. BMJ 1995;310:830–3.

[73] Carolei A, Marini C, De Matteis G, et al. History of migraine and risk of cerebral ischaemia in young adults. Lancet 1996;347:1503–6.

[74] Chang CL, Donaghy M, Poulter N, et al. Migraine and stroke in young women: case-control study. BMJ 1999;318:13–8.

[75] World Health Organization. Improving access to quality care in family planning: medical eligibility criteria for contraceptive use. Geneva (Switzerland): World Health Organization; 2004. p. 75–87.

[76] Winkler U. Effects of progestins on cardiovascular diseases: the haemostatic system. Hum Reprod Update 1999;5:200.

[77] American College of Obstetricians and Gynecologists. Hormonal contraception. ACOG Technical Bulletin. Washington (DC): ACOG; 1994. p. 198.

[78] van Hooff M, et al. The use of oral contraceptives by adolescents for contraception, menstrual cycle problems or acne. Acta Obstet Gynecol Scand 1998;77:898–904.

ELSEVIER
SAUNDERS

ADOLESCENT
MEDICINE
CLINICS

Adolesc Med 16 (2005) 553–567

Progestin Only Contraceptives and Their Use in Adolescents: Clinical Options and Medical Indications

Amy M. Burkett, MD, Geri D. Hewitt, MD*

The Ohio State University College of Medicine and School of Public Health, 516 Means Hall, 1654 Upham Drive, Columbus, OH 43210, USA

This article reviews progestin only contraceptives and their use in adolescent women. Young women requiring hormonal contraceptives for birth control or medical indications may prefer or require a nonestrogen containing product. This article reviews the products currently available, those soon to be released, and those under development. Many relatively common clinical situations preclude the use of estrogen-containing contraceptives or combination hormonal contraceptives, and those also will be outlined.

Progestin only hormonal contraceptives

Depot medroxyprogesterone acetate

Depot medroxyprogesterone acetate (DMPA) is discussed in detail in another section, but warrants brief mention here because it is used so widely. DMPA is given intramuscularly every 12 weeks and works by suppressing the luteinizing hormone (LH) surge and inhibiting ovulation [1]. Failure rate is less than 1% over 1 year of perfect use, but with typical use, the failure rate is 3% [2]. The most commonly experienced adverse effect is menstrual irregularity, including amenorrhea [1]. Other potential adverse effects include depression, weight gain, and a longer interval of return to baseline fertility when compared with oral

---

* Corresponding author.

E-mail address: hewitt-2@medctr.osu.edu (G.D. Hewitt).

1547-3368/05/$ – see front matter © 2005 Elsevier Inc. All rights reserved.
doi:10.1016/j.admecli.2005.05.010   *adolescent.theclinics.com*

contraceptives [3]. There is also increasing concern regarding bone mineral density loss with use in patients younger than 14 and with long-term use. This concern has led the manufacturer to change the package insert to limit the duration of use to 2 years unless no other hormonal contraceptive method is available [4,5].

Progestin only pills

Progestin only pills come in three separate formulations in the United States. Micronor and Nor-QD each contain 0.35 mg of norethindrone; Ovrette contains 0.075 mg of norgestrel. Progestin only pills are all active pills, with no inert pills or placebos, and they need to be taken daily, at the same time (Table 1) [1]. This required level of diligence can be a challenging obstacle for adolescent use. Progestin only pills have a perfect use failure rate of 0.3%. Because it must be taken at the same time every day, its typical use failure rate is upwards of 10% [2]. The progestin only pill works by suppressing ovulation, thickening cervical mucus, and causing atrophy of the endometrium [1,6], thus creating an inhospitable uterine environment to the sperm and ovum. Like all oral contraceptives, the progestin only pill will not disrupt an implanted pregnancy, cause miscarriage, or birth defects [7]. Adverse effects include amenorrhea, intermenstrual spotting, and altered menstrual flow. Up to one-third of women who are using these pills while not lactating will experience an abnormal bleeding pattern. Patients should be counseled regarding longer cycles and intermenstrual spotting, as these are the most common complaints leading to discontinuation. Patients using them while lactating are more likely to experience amenorrhea. This effect likely is related to lactational amenorrhea and is well tolerated, as the discontinuation rate in the lactating population is lower. Although menstrual irregularities may be more common in nonlactating patients using progestin only pills compared with estrogen-containing pills, headaches and breast tenderness are less common [6].

Table 1
Difference between progestin-only and combined hormonal contraceptives

Characteristic	Progestin-only contraceptives	Combination hormonal contraceptives
Contains estrogen	No	Yes
Pill-free interval or placebo pills	No	Yes
Amenorrhea	Often	Rare
Suppresses ovulation	Yes	Yes
Alters cervical mucus	Yes	Yes

Data from A pocket guide to managing contraception. Tiger (GA): Bridging the Gap Foundation; 2004. p. 120–35.

Implanon

Implanon is a plastic polymer rod implant containing etonogestestrel that is available only in Europe [8], but it has received Food and Drug Administration (FDA) approval [9] and will to be released in the United States soon [1]. Implanon is inserted by a health care professional underneath the skin to provide long-term (up to 3 years) contraception [8]. Like other forms of hormonal contraception, the mechanism of action with the contraceptive rod is inhibition of ovulation [1]. Implanon is an excellent hormonal contraceptive option for young women, because there is little need for ongoing patient compliance after insertion, and the pregnancy rate is remarkably low. An initial study published in 1999 reported no pregnancies in its study population, which included over 1200 woman-years. Norplant was a contraceptive rod system with six silastic rods containing levonorgestrel. When inserted under the skin, it was effective for up to 5 years [10]. Researchers feel comfortable projecting Implanon's contraceptive efficacy to be comparable to Norplant's, which had a 0% to 0.6% failure rate in the first 3 years of use and a 0.6% to 1% failure rate at 5 years of use [11,12]. Implanon has distinct advantages over Norplant directly related to its development into a single rod with a different plastic polymer that will allow greater ease of insertion and removal [8].

Implants are well accepted by women. In a study looking specifically at an adolescent population, 93% were satisfied with Norplant. Implanon should be as well accepted as Norplant or even more so given its ease of insertion and removal. Adolescents tend to choose an implant after a contraceptive failure, particularly one resulting in pregnancy. They also switch to an implant when they experience adverse effects from other methods. Some simply choose implants because they like the device's convenience and ease of use [13]. Patients need to be counseled to expect altered bleeding patterns ranging from amenorrhea to prolonged and heavy menstrual flow; these are the most common reasons sited for early removal of Implanon. Other reasons sited include desired pregnancy, worsening of acne, weight gain [10], breast tenderness, and headache [14]. Most adverse effects experienced by patients using Implanon were not bothersome enough for the patient to have the device removed [14].

Emergency contraception

Up to 30% of patients have never heard of emergency contraception, and only 10% know how to obtain it [15]. Emergency contraception is described in detail elsewhere in this issue; this article briefly describes the progestin only method. There are three common pill regimens available, the Yuzpe Method, Plan B, and low-dose mifepristone [16,17]. Plan B is the progestin only method of emergency contraception. It contains two 0.75 mg doses of levonorgestrel, which are to be taken 12 hours apart. It is highly effective in preventing pregnancy after an act of unprotected intercourse. When used in the first 24 hours after unprotected intercourse, one study found only 2 of 450 women became pregnant.

Although the method is most effective in the first 24 hours, it can be used up to 72 hours after unprotected intercourse [18]. Emergency contraception can be very helpful to young women who experience rape, sexual abuse, contraceptive failure, or a spontaneous, unpredictable sexual encounter where contraception was not used or planned for in advance. Although progestin only emergency contraception will not harm an existing pregnancy, the only contraindication to its use is pregnancy [7]. Therefore if a clinician is contacted regarding a patient's need for emergency contraception, they can simply have the patient do a home urine pregnancy test and, if negative, call in a prescription to a local pharmacy for "Plan B, to use as directed." It is important to initiate the therapy as soon as possible after the act of intercourse. The young woman can follow up in the office at an appropriate interval for contraception counseling, sexually transmitted infection (STI) testing, and a follow-up pregnancy test. Adverse effects are less common with plan B than the other methods, but they include nausea, vomiting, breast tenderness [18], and irregular bleeding patterns [19]. These patterns include spotting, shortened interval to menses, and lighter or heavier menses [19]. Teenagers should not mistake spotting for a light menses, as spotting does not always indicate success of emergency contraception [18,19]. Studies show that adolescents who are given emergency contraception before a method failure (advance provision) are more likely to use it than those who have to obtain it after unprotected intercourse has occurred. These data support providing all sexually active adolescents prescriptions for emergency contraception [20].

Intrauterine devices

Intrauterine devices (IUDs) have a long and mixed history as contraception in the United States, much of which stems from the now obsolete Dalkon Shield [21]. IUDs often are not considered a viable method of contraception in the adolescent population, but research shows that in a carefully screened population, the device can be successful. Adolescents should be mutually monogamous, placing them at low risk for STIs. They do not have to be parous, but there is a higher expulsion rate in the nulliparous patient [22]. The Mirena IUD (Table 2) contains a progestin. It works by slowing releasing levonorgestrel into the

Table 2
Comparison of copper and progestin containing intrauterine devices

Characteristic	Copper IUD	Progestin IUD
Mechanism of action	Spermicidal	Spermicidal
Active ingredient	Copper	Levonorgestrel
Bleeding pattern	Unchanged to heavier menses	Unchanged to lighter menses
Duration of use	10 years	5 years
FDA approval with lactation	Yes	No

FEI women's health. ParaGard patient information booklet. FEI women's health 2003. Available at: http://www.paragard.com/images/Package-Insert.pdf. Accessed November 18, 2004.
Data from Mirena. Available at: www.fda.gov/cder/foi/nda/2000/21-225/pdf_Mirena_Prntlbl.pdf. Accessed October 31, 2004.

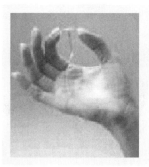

ParaGard is made of soft, white plastic, in the shape of a small "T." It's 1 3/8 inches long, with small amounts of copper wrapped around the stem and arms. The copper enhances the effectiveness of ParaGard.

Fig. 1. ParaGard is made of soft white plastic in the shape of a small "T." It is 1.375 inches long, with small amounts of copper wrapped around the stem and arms. The copper enhances effectiveness. (*From* www.paragard.com.)

endometrial cavity over a 5-year period and has a failure rate of 0.1% [2]. The device works locally, causing thickened cervical mucus and an atrophic endometrium. This environment is toxic to sperm because of local inflammation [23]. The ParaGard IUD is not hormonally active but contains copper, again causing endometrial inflammation that is toxic to sperm (Fig. 1). Both IUDs are spermicidal. The copper IUD is effective for up to 10 years after insertion [24] and has a failure rate of 0.8% per year with typical use [2]. Most women experience a decrease in menstrual bleeding while using the Mirena IUD, but bleeding profiles when using the nonhormonally active IUD can be heavier than a patient's preinsertion menses [24]. Because both devices are very effective in preventing pregnancy, the rate of ectopic pregnancy is lower than that seen in the general population [24,25]. The Mirena IUD is not recommended for patients with a history of ectopic pregnancy, as these patients were not included in the clinical trials [25]. Complications associated with IUDs include uterine perforation during insertion, insertion-related endometritis [24], and increased dysmenorrhea that usually responds to nonsteroidal anti-inflammatory drugs (NSAIDs). The most common reasons patients request IUD removal are bleeding and pain [22]. Antibiotic prophylaxis at the time of insertion is recommended only for patients who receive prophylaxis for other procedures, such as dental work [24].

Future methods

Researchers continue to strive for hormonal contraception that is simple, effective, and user friendly. To that end, there are efforts to create an implant that is biodegradable when exposed to body fluids. Such a device is Capronor, a capsule consisting of levonorgestrel, which slowly dissolves. A second device consisting of four to five pellets of norethindrone is in early development [1,2]. If successful, both devices would alleviate the uncomfortable process of removing a device, while still providing the long-term, effective, and effortless contraception many adolescents desire.

Vaginal rings as alternative delivery system are receiving attention also. A combination contraceptive ring containing both estrogen and progestin is already available in the United States. A progestin only ring is available in South America, indicated currently only for use during lactation. Further use and development of progestin only rings had been halted in the 1980s because of concern over adverse lipid profiles and vaginal lesions. There is a phase II trial underway looking at a nestorone-containing ring that could stay in place for 6 to 12 months in lactating women [26].

Clinical indications for progestin only contraceptives

Lactation

Some adolescent mothers are very interested in breastfeeding, and with appropriate education and support, they are successful at breastfeeding exclusively. Most clinicians are familiar with the use of the progestin only contraceptive methods during lactation. Because estrogen-containing hormonal contraceptives affect breast milk production, progestin only options are the preferred choice. Controversy exists regarding when to initiate progestin only contraceptives in the postpartum period. Most authorities, including the National Medical Community of Planned Parenthood Federation, agree that it is acceptable to begin them immediately postpartum, but the World Health Organization (WHO) and International Planned Parenthood Federation recommend waiting until 6 weeks postpartum [27]. Some clinicians prefer to wait until the 6 week postpartum visit to decrease the likelihood of abnormal bleeding [28] and to secure lactogenesis [29]. The authors' practice has been to initiate progestin contraceptives before discharge from the hospital for several reasons. First, a significant proportion of teen mothers in their practice have initiated sexual activity before their 6-week follow-up appointment. Second, few of their young mothers breastfeed ex-

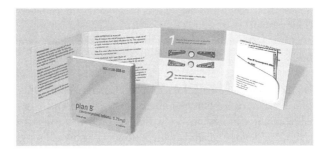

Fig. 2. Plan B. (*From* http://ec.princeton.edu/Pills/planb.html.)

clusively, and third, compliance at the 6-week postpartum examination is often less than 100%. DMPA, progestin only pills, and contraceptive rods can be initiated before discharge from the hospital (Fig. 2). The progestin IUD is not approved by the FDA for use in lactating women [25]. Latino women with gestational diabetes are at increased risk of developing diabetes in the first year after delivery if they are lactating and using progestin only pills [30]. Although this is not a contraindication to using progestin only pills in this population, it emphasizes the need for diabetes screening during this period (Fig. 3).

Gynecologic disorders

Often times an adolescent may present to the pediatrician with gynecologic complaints, including dysmenorrhea, pelvic pain associated with endometriosis, polycystic ovarian syndrome, and anovulatory bleeding. Progestin only contraceptives may play a role in managing these common gynecologic complaints.

Medical problems

Although most adolescent women are healthy and without medical risk factors or disease, there are numerous health problems that can preclude a young woman from using estrogen-containing birth control methods (Table 3) [7,31]. Approximately 10% of adolescents are diagnosed with a major medical condition by the time they are 18 [32]. Therefore, practitioners should screen their patients for personal and family medical conditions that could affect their contraceptive choice. Screening questions should include personal or family history of neurological disorders, cardiovascular disease, sickle cell anemia, liver dysfunction, and diabetes. It should be noted that there are no medical conditions that preclude the use of progestin only emergency contraception [7].

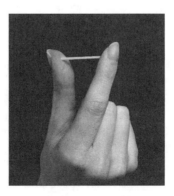

Fig. 3. The implantable contraceptive rod.

Table 3
Medical conditions and their impact on hormonal contraceptive choice

Medical conditions	Progestin-only contraceptives	Combination hormonal contraceptives
Asymptomatic MVP	Yes	Yes
Symptomatic MVP	Yes	No
MVP associated with smoking, history of thromboembolism, or hypercoaguable disorders	Yes	No
Uncomplicated valvular disorders	Yes	Yes
Complicated valvular disorders	Yes	No
Hypertension	Yes	No
Hypertension limited to pregnancy	Yes	Yes
Uncontrolled hypertension	Yes (excluding depo-MPA)	No
Multiple cardiac risk factors	Yes (excluding depo-MPA)	No
Congenital heart disease	Yes	No
Acute DVT or PE	No	No
Resolved DVT or PE	Yes	No
Family history of DVT or PE	Yes	Yes
Inherited thrombogenic disorders	Yes	No
Acquired hypercoaguable disorders	Yes	No
Uncontrolled dyslipidemia with LDL >160	Yes	Yes
Nonmigrainous headaches	Yes	Yes
Migrainous heachaches without aura	Yes	Yes
Migrainous headache with aura >1 hour	Yes	No
Migrainous headaches with neurologic symptoms	Yes	No
Migrainous headaches with stroke risk factors	Yes	No
Seizure disorder	Yes	Yes
Diabetes	Yes	Yes
Diabetes with end organ damage	Yes	No
Sickle cell disease	Yes	Yes
Active hepatitis	No	No
Chronic hepatitis	Yes	No
Liver tumors	Yes	No
Mild cirrhosis	Yes	No
Decompensated cirrhosis	No	No
Active gallbladder disease	Yes	No
History of cholecystectomy	Yes	Yes
Wilson's disease	Yes	No
Liver transplant	Yes	Yes

Data from Curtis KM, Gaffield ME, Mohllajee AP, et al. Medical eligibility criteria for contraceptive use. 3rd edition. Geneva (Switzerland): World Health Organization; 2004.
Sullivan JM, Lobo RA. Considerations for contraception in women with cardiovascular disorders. AJOG 1993;168(6S):2006–11.
Heroux K. Contraceptive choices in medically ill adolescents. Semin Reprod Med 2003;21(4):389–98.
American College of Obstetricians and Gynecologists. 2004 Compendium of selected publications. Washington (DC): American College of Obstetricians and Gynecologists; 2004.
Evans RW, Lipton RB. Topics in migraine management: a survey of headache specialists highlights some controversies. Neurologic Clinics 2001;19(1).
Neinstein L. Contraception in women with special medical needs. Compr Ther 1998;24(5):229–50.
Connolly TJ, Zuckerman AL. Contraception in the patient with liver disease. Semin Perinatol 1999;22(2):178–82.

Cardiovascular disease

Adolescents should be asked about cardiac disorders and cardiovascular risk factors when considering hormonal contraception. These risk factors include [34]:

- Smoking
- Diabetes
- Hypertension
- Family history of premature cardiac events
- History of cerebral vascular accident
- Low high-density lipoprotein (HDL) (less than 35)
- Elevated triglycerides (greater than 250)
- Elevated low-density lipoprotein (LDL) (greater than 160)
- Cardiac anomaly

Young women may not remember the specific disease entity, but one can screen for medication use, emergency room visits for chest pain, use of antibiotics during dental procedures, chest surgery, or a history of having an echocardiogram. Young women with asymptomatic mitral valve prolapse (MVP) can use combination hormonal contraception safely [7,33]. Patients with symptomatic MVP or MVP associated with smoking, history of thromboembolic events, or coagulopathy should not use combination hormonal contraception but can use progestin only birth control methods safely [33]. Teenagers with other uncomplicated cardiac valvular syndromes may use combination hormonal contraceptives [7]. Cardiac valvular syndromes complicated by pulmonary hypertension, risk of atrial fibrillation, or history of subacute bacterial endocarditis preclude the use of combination hormonal contraceptives. These patients can use progestin only methods safely [7]. Patients with valvular disease other than asymptomatic MVP require antibiotic prophylaxis against bacterial endocarditis at the time of IUD insertion [7,33].

Current WHO recommendations suggest that women with hypertension should avoid combination hormonal contraception and would be served better with the use of progestin only contraceptive methods. Young women with a history of hypertension limited to pregnancy can use combination hormonal contraception safely. Patients with uncontrolled hypertension (systolic blood pressure greater than or equal to 160 or diastolic blood pressure greater than or equal to 100) or multiple cardiac risk factors should avoid DMPA, but they may use any other progestin only methods safely [7].

More infants born with cardiac anomalies are living well into their reproductive years and require counseling about choosing acceptable methods of birth control. Pregnancy can expose these patients to significant risk of maternal morbidity and mortality. Many of these disorders, even when repaired, are complicated with other cardiac diseases, which preclude the use of combination hormonal contraceptives. Although there is an array of cardiac syndromes, generally the use of progestin only contraceptive methods is safe [32]. Both IUDs are also an acceptable choice in this patient population [7,32].

Box 1. Inherited hypercoagulable disorders

Antithrombin deficiency
Abnormalities in protein C and protein S system

- Protein C deficiency
- Protein S deficiency
- Abnormal thrombomodulin

Resistance to activated C protein (factor V Leiden)
Hyperprothrombinemia (prothrombin variant G20210A)
Hyperhomocystinemia
Dysfibrinogenemia
Abnormalities in fibrinolytic system

- Hypo- or dysplasminogenemis
- Elevated plasminogen activator inhibitor
- Decreased tissue plasminogen activator

Heparin cofactor II deficiency
Elevated histidine-rich glycoprotein
Factor XII deficiency

(*Reprinted from* Rao AK, Sheth S, Kaplan R. Inherited coagulable states. Vasc Med 1997;2(4):314; with permission.)

Teenagers with an active or resolved DVT (deep vein thrombosis) or PE (pulmonary embolus) cannot use combination hormonal contraceptives. In the patient with an active DVT or PE, progestin only methods should be avoided also, but they can be used safely after resolution of the acute event. Family history of DVT or PE does not preclude a teenager from using combined hormonal contraceptive methods unless a clotting disorder also was diagnosed [7].

Patients diagnosed with hereditary thrombogenic mutations (Box 1) should avoid combination hormonal contraceptives, but they can use all types of progestin only methods safely. Current WHO recommendations maintain that routine screening tests for thrombogenic disorders are not required before prescribing combination hormonal contraceptives [7]. If a young woman reports a family history of acute thromboembolic events or thrombogenic mutations, however, appropriate screening tests should be done [7,34]. These tests include [36] (personal communication with P. Samuels, MD, December 2004):

- Genetic testing for factor V Leiden
- Genetic testing for prothrombin gene 20210A
- Plasma levels of protein C, protein S, antithrombin

- PT/INR
- PTT
- Plasma levels of homocysteine (if elevated, consider genetic testing for methyleneterahydrofolate reductase homozygosity and cystathionine β-synthase deficiency

The most prevalent disorder diagnosed is factor V Leiden mutation, affecting 7% of Caucasians [34]. Young patients with a personal history of thrombosis in less common places or without trauma should be screened for the acquired hypercoagulable disorders in addition to the heritable thrombogenic disorders. The American College of Obstetrics and Gynecology (ACOG) specifically suggests screening for antiphospholipid antibodies and anticardiolipin antibodies in this patient population, as these disorders can complicate pregnancy outcomes and are a contraindication to combination hormonal contraception [35]. In adolescents diagnosed with hypercoagulable disorders progestin only birth control methods can be used safely so long as the patient does not currently have a DVT or pulmonary embolus (PE). Combined hormonal contraceptive methods should be avoided [7].

The WHO does not recommend routine lipid profile screening in healthy adolescents before prescribing combination hormonal contraception [7]. If a screening lipid profile is done for other reasons and identifies a dyslipidemia, there are specific recommendations for the use of hormonal contraception. Adolescents with controlled dyslipidemias have no limitations on their contraceptive choice as estrogens have a positive effect on HDL and LDL. If a young woman has an LDL greater than 160 or other cardiac risk factors, however, she should not use combined hormonal contraception, because estrogens elevate triglycerides [32]. These patients may use progestin only methods safely [32,36]. Patients with dyslipidemias on combination hormonal contraceptives should have their lipid profiles followed closely [32].

Neurologic conditions

Screening questions for neurological disorders should focus on headaches and seizures. Teenagers with nonmigrainous or migrainous headaches without aura are not limited from use of combined hormonal contraceptives [7,37,38]. Migraines with aura lasting longer than 1 hour or accompanied by neurological symptoms such as numbness, weakness, or tingling preclude the use of combined hormonal contraceptives. Additionally if patients with migraines have stroke risk factors, they should not use combined hormonal contraceptives [31,37,38]. If a young woman begins to experience auras while using a progestin only method, it should be discontinued [7].

Young women with seizure disorders need reliable contraception because of the teratogenicity of most anticonvulsants [31]. No seizure disorder precludes the use of combined hormonal contraception. Many anticonvulsants, however, decrease the efficacy of combined and progestin only hormonal contraception, primarily through enhanced liver activity [7,31]. DMPA is the least affected by this process, likely because the serum concentrations are higher compared with other methods [31]. Although some clinicians increase the dose of the hormonal contraceptive prescribed in patients taking anticonvulsants, it is uncertain whether this will increase its efficacy [7]. Patients on anticonvulsants may choose barrier methods and either IUD, as their efficacy is not affected by liver metabolism.

Diabetes

Adolescents with type 1, type 2, or a history of gestational diabetes mellitus can use any method of hormonal contraception safely unless there is end organ damage (nephropathy, retinopathy, or vascular disease). The presence of end organ damage precludes the use of combined hormonal methods, but these patients can use progestin only birth control methods, barrier methods, or either IUD safely [7,38]. Young mothers who had gestational diabetes should be screened for impaired glucose tolerance after delivery [39]. All diabetic women should be counseled about the importance of glycemic control, because hyperglycemia is related directly to an increased risk of birth defects. This illustrates the need for glycemic control when attempting conception and emphasizes the need for good, reliable contraception in patients with diabetes [40].

Sickle cell disease

Sickle cell disease is not a contraindication to the use of combined hormonal contraceptives. Small controlled trials suggest that patients using DMPA experience fewer crises, and therefore ACOG considers it the method of choice in these patients [38].

Hepatobiliary disease

Some types of gallbladder and liver disease preclude the use of hormonal contraceptives. When screening for these disorders, clinicians should ask about jaundice after the newborn period, history of cholecystectomy, presence of gallbladder disease, medically imposed dietary restrictions, intravenous drug abuse, current and past sexual practices, and history of blood transfusion before 1992 or transfusion of clotting factors before 1987 [41]. Active hepatitis precludes the use of all hormonal contraceptives, but these patients may use barrier methods and copper IUDs. Patients with chronic hepatitis can use progestin only options, barrier methods, and both IUDs. Adolescents with liver tumors or mild cirrhosis should not use combined hormonal contraceptives, as they can exacerbate these disorders. These patients can use progestin only methods safely [7,42]. Young women with decompensated cirrhosis should avoid all hormonal contraception but may consider a copper IUD [7]. Patients with active gallbladder disease are candidates for progestin birth control, but they should not use combination hormonal contraceptives until after cholecystectomy [7]. Adolescents with Wilson's disease should avoid the copper IUD and combination hormonal contraceptives but may use progestin methods safely. Any young woman who has received a liver transplant can use the progestin only methods safely, but the use of combined hormonal contraception is controversial. Patients taking combined hormonal contraceptives need to have liver function tests and cyclosporine levels monitored closely. Use of IUDs in liver transplant patients is also controversial because of their immunosuppression, which may cause an increased risk of ascending infection. There is also concern that the immunosuppressive agents may lessen the efficacy of the copper IUD, as its affects are thought to be exerted partially through the immune system [42].

Patient choice

Patient lifestyle always plays a role in the choice of contraceptive. Although choosing a contraceptive method, counseling adolescents, and sexual activity are addressed elsewhere in greater detail, it should be noted that DMPA and implantable devices often are chosen by young women simply because of ease of use. These methods do not require the adolescent to remember a pill every day, and they provide discreet, long-term contraception with minimal hassle.

Summary

Most adolescents are healthy and can use combined hormonal contraception safely. In clinical situations that preclude the use of these agents, the patient often can be served well by a progestin only method. The progestin only contraceptive options include pills, a long acting intramuscular injection, an implant, and a progestin IUD. Although the options vary in their efficacy, they are generally safe and well tolerated by adolescents. In particular, implants are suited well for adolescent use because of their low need for compliance and high efficacy and continuation rates. Pregnancy is the only contraindication to progestin only emergency contraception, and studies show advanced provision enhances its appropriate use in the adolescent population.

Acknowledgments

The authors would like to thank Ms. Laura Trout-Molton for her help in preparation of the final manuscript and Ms. Megan Dailey for her assistance in accessing numerous reference articles.

References

[1] Hatcher RA, Ziemann M, Cwiak C, et al. Progestin only contraceptives. In: A pocket guide to managing contraception. Tiger (GA): Bridging the Gap Foundation; 2004.

[2] Trussell J. Contraceptive failure in the United States. Contraception 2004;70:89–96.

[3] Hewitt G, Cromer B. Update in adolescent contraception. Obstet Gynecol Clin North Am 2000; 27(1):143–62.

[4] Pfizer. Additional prescribing information for Depo-Provera. Available at: http://www.pfizer. com/download/uspi_depo_provera_contraceptive.pdf. Accessed November 18, 2004.

[5] Pharmacia. Depo-Provera Contraceptive Injection (product insert). Pharmacia-Upjohn Company. 2004.

[6] Kovacs G. Progestogen only pills and bleeding disturbances. Hum Reprod 1996;11(2S): 20–3.

[7] Curtis KM, Gaffield ME, Mohllajee AP, et al. Medical eligibility criteria for contraceptive use. 3rd edition. Geneva (Switzerland): World Health Organization; 2004.

[8] Mishell Jr DR. State of the art of hormonal contraception: an overview. AJOG 2004;190(4):S1–4.

[9] Organon's contraceptive Implanon receives approvable status from the FDA USA Page. Available at: http://www.organon-usa.com/news/2004_11_04_implanon_approved_by_fda.asp. Accessed November 12, 2004.

[10] Croxatto H. Progestin implants for female contraception. Contraception 2002;65:15–9.

[11] Croxatto HB, Urbansek J, Massai R, et al. A multi-centre efficacy and safety study of the single contraceptive implant Implanon. Hum Reprod 1999;14(4):976–81.

[12] Mechstroth KR, Darney PD. Implant contraception. Semin Reprod Med 2001;19(4):339–54.

[13] Berenson AB, Wiemann CM. Use of levorgestrel implants versus oral contraceptives in adolescence: a case-control study. AJOG 1995;172(4):1128–37.

[14] Urbancsek J. An integrated analysis of nonmenstrual adverse events with Implanon. Contraception 1998;58:109S–15S.

[15] Trussell J, Ellertson C. Efficacy of emergency contraception. Fertility Control Reviews 1995;4: 8–11.

[16] Von Hertzen H, Piaggo G, Ding J, et al. Low-dose mifepristone and two regimens of levonorgestrel for emergency contraception: a WHO multi-centre randomized trial. Lancet 2002; 360:1803–10.

[17] Hatcher RA, Ziemann M, Cwiak C. Emergency contraception. In: A pocket guide to managing contraception. Tiger (GA): Bridging the Gap Foundation; 2004. p. 73–83.

[18] Task Force on Postovulatory Methods of Fertility Regulation. Randomised controlled trial of levonorgestrel versus Yuzpe regimen of combined oral contraceptives for emergency birth control. Lancet 1998;352:428–33.

[19] Webb A, Scochet T, Bigrigg A, et al. Effect of hormonal emergency contraception on bleeding patterns. Contraception 2004;60:133–5.

[20] Gold MA, Wolford JE, Smith KA, et al. The effects of advance provision on emergency contraception on adolescent women's sexual and contraceptive behaviors. J Pediatr Adolesc Gynecol 2004;17:87–96.

[21] Hubacher D. The checkered history and bright future of intrauterine contraception in the United States. Perspect Sex Reprod Health 2002;34(2):98–103.

[22] Sulak PJ. Intrauterine device practice guidelines: patient types. Contraception 1998;5:55S–8S.

[23] Shulman LP, Nelson AL, Darney PD. Recent developments in hormone delivery systems. AJOG 2004;190(4S):S39–48.

[24] Mishell Jr DR. Intrauterine devices: mechanisms of action, safety, and efficacy. Contraception 1998;58:45S–53S.

[25] Mirena. Available at: www.fda.gov/cder/foi/nda/2000/21-225/pdf_Mirena_Prntlbl.pdf. Accessed October 31, 2004.

[26] Johansson EDB, Sitruk-Ware R. New delivery systems in contraception: vaginal rings. AJOG 2004;190(4S):S54–9.

[27] Hatcher RA, Ziemann M, Cwiak C, et al. Breastfeeding and contraceptive decisions. In: A pocket guide to managing contraception. Tiger (GA): Bridging the Gap Foundation; 2004. p. 46.

[28] Hawkins DF, Elder MG. Human fertility control, theory and practice. London: (Butterworth); 1979.

[29] Kennedy KI, Short RV, Tully MR. Premature introduction of progestin only methods during lactation. Contraception 1997;55:347–50.

[30] Kjos SL, Peters RK, Xianq A, et al. Contraception and the risk of type 2 diabetes mellitus in Latina women with prior gestational diabetes mellitus. JAMA 1998;280:533–8.

[31] Neinstein L. Contraception in women with special medical needs. Compr Ther 1998;24(5): 229–50.

[32] Heroux K. Contraceptive choices in medically ill adolescents. Semin Reprod Med 2003;21(4): 389–98.

[33] Sullivan JM, Lobo RA. Considerations for contraception in women with cardiovascular disorders. AJOG 1993;168(6S):2006–11.

[34] Rao AK, Sheth S, Kaplan R. Inherited hypercoagulable states. Vasc Med 1997;2(4):313–20.

[35] American College of Obstetricians and Gynecologists. ACOG Educational Bulletin 224: antiphospholipid syndrome, February 1998. In: 2004 Compendium of selected publications. Washington (DC): ACOG; 2004. p. 149–58.

[36] Knopp R, LaRosa JC, Burkman Jr T. Contraception and Dyslipidemia. AJOG 1993;168(6S): 1994–2005.

[37] Evans RW, Lipton RB. Topics in migraine management: A survey of headache specialists highlights some controversies. Neurologic Clinics 2001;19(1) NP. Available at http://home. mdconsult.com/das/article/body/41197932-2.

[38] American College of Obstetricians and Gynecologists. ACOG Practice Bulletin 18: The use of hormonal contraception in women with coexisting medical conditions, July 2004. In 2004 Compendium of Selected Publications. Washington DC: ACOG; 2004. p. 674–87.

[39] American College of Obstetricians and Gynecologists. ACOG Practice Bulletin 30: Gestational Diabetes, September 2001. In 2004 Compendium of Selected Publications. Washington DC: ACOG; 2004. p. 398–411.

[40] Mestman JH, Schmidt-Sarosi C. Diabetes mellitus and fertility control: contraception management issues. AJOG 1993;168(6S):2012–20.

[41] Adams PC, Arthur MJ, Boyer TD, et al. Screening in liver disease: report of an AASLD clinical workshop. Hepatology 2004;39(5):1204–12.

[42] Connolly TJ, Zuckerman AL. Contraception in the patient with liver disease. Semin Perinatol 1999;22(2):178–82.

ELSEVIER
SAUNDERS

ADOLESCENT
MEDICINE
CLINICS

Adolesc Med 16 (2005) 569–584

Depot Medroxyprogesterone Acetate: Implications for Weight Status and Bone Mineral Density in the Adolescent Female

Andrea E. Bonny, MD[a,b,*], Laura S. Harkness, PhD[a,b], Barbara A. Cromer, MD[a,b]

[a]Case Western Reserve University School of Medicine, 10900 Euclid Avenue, Cleveland, OH 44106, USA
[b]Division of Adolescent Medicine, MetroHealth Medical Center, 2500 MetroHealth Drive, Cleveland, OH 44109, USA

Since its introduction in the 1970s, depot medroxyprogesterone acetate (DMPA) has endured medical and political controversy, causing its delayed approval as a contraceptive agent in the United States for almost 20 years [1]. Its continued use and success, despite such controversy, are because of its unique features and strengths as a contraceptive agent [2]. DMPA is a progestin-only contraceptive given intramuscularly every 3 months. It is extremely effective (less than 1% annual failure rate), obviates the need for daily pill compliance, and can be used privately [2]. As such, DMPA has many features that are clinically appealing for use in adolescents. It is estimated that 1 million adolescent girls between the ages of 15 and 19 use DMPA as their contraceptive method [3]. The decreased incidence of adolescent pregnancy over the past decade has been attributed, in part, to the increased use of DMPA [4].

New questions, however, have emerged regarding DMPA use in adolescents and potential important adverse effects. Weight gain, although not a new concern, remains a persistent issue for patients and clinicians, and new literature suggests the potential for exaggerated weight gain in obese adolescents [5–8] and ab-

---

* Corresponding author. Department of Pediatrics, MetroHealth Medical Center, 2500 Metro-Health Drive, Cleveland, OH 44109.
  E-mail address: abonny@metrohealth.org (A.E. Bonny).

1547-3368/05/$ – see front matter © 2005 Elsevier Inc. All rights reserved.
doi:10.1016/j.admecli.2005.05.006   *adolescent.theclinics.com*

normal increases in adiposity in all adolescents [9]. In light of the current epidemic of adolescent obesity, these issues are of particular relevance.

Concern has developed regarding DMPA use and potential negative impact on bone mineral density (BMD). In November 2004, the Food and Drug Administration (FDA) issued a black box warning regarding DMPA use and potential effects on bone [10]. In its warning, the FDA stated that "women who use DMPA may lose significant BMD. Bone loss is greater with increasing duration of use and may not be completely reversible. DMPA should be used as a long-term birth control method (eg, longer than 2 years) only if other birth control methods are inadequate." The FDA also noted in its warning that "it is unknown if use of DMPA during adolescence or early adulthood will reduce peak bone mass and increase the risk for osteoporotic fracture in later life." Hence, the implications of DMPA use in adolescence for adult bone health remain unclear.

As the controversy about the use of DMPA is played out, it is done in the context of the United States having the highest rate of adolescent pregnancy in the industrialized world [11,12]. A need for effective contraception for the sexually active adolescent remains, and DMPA is a valuable contraceptive tool for this population. Although contraceptive options are increasing, including the advent of the transdermal patch [13] and continuous oral contraceptives [14], DMPA, with its ease of use and long-acting potential, remains an ideal contraceptive for adolescents. It is important, therefore, to critically evaluate the current research on DMPA use in adolescents.

This article examines the literature regarding DMPA use in adolescents with respect to weight gain and BMD and considers potential implications for current clinical practice.

Depot medroxyprogesterone acetate and weight

Weight gain from DMPA is not a new clinical concern. Weight gain has been reported in up to 54% of adolescents receiving DMPA contraception [15] and is cited as the primary reason for method discontinuation by 41% of adolescents who use this method [16]. Nearly 33% of adolescents who begin DMPA do not receive a second injection at 3 months, and 75% discontinue use by 12 months [17]. Only 9% of adolescents who discontinue because of weight gain will restart DMPA, compared with 80% who discontinue owing to missed appointments [17].

Despite anecdotal complaints about weight gain among adolescent females on DMPA and frequently documented effects of weight gain on DMPA continuation, weight gain is not a universal finding in research studies. A summary of the literature examining DMPA and weight gain among adolescents is shown in Table 1. Most studies are limited by lack of prospective data or adequate control groups. For example, Moore and colleagues conducted a retrospective chart review of 150 women (age: 15 to 30 years) on DMPA, oral contraceptives, or contraceptive implants [18]. At 1 year of use, the authors found no significant weight gain in any group. Because women experiencing weight gain are more likely to discontinue their contraceptive method, the retrospective nature of this study could bias results. In addition, the authors did not report the race or ethnicity of their study subjects.

In four other retrospective studies examining DMPA use and weight in adolescents, significant associations with weight were found [5,6,17,19]. Templeman and colleagues compared two groups of adolescent females on DMPA [19]. Group 1 consisted of 73 adolescents (mean age: 14.8 years) from a state-funded pregnancy prevention clinic who received DMPA injections at 3-month intervals. Group 2 consisted of 60 adolescents (mean age: 15.6 years) from a private clinic who received DMPA monthly for 3 months and then converted to standard 3-month injection dosing. There was statistically significant ($P = .001$) weight gain in both groups at 12 months (Group 1: 9.8 lbs; Group 2: 7.7 lbs). No adolescents off hormonal contraception were available for comparison.

In two retrospective studies, it was reported that being overweight at initiation of DMPA resulted in greater weight gain. Risser and colleagues compared 130 adolescents (age: 13 to 19 years) on DMPA or oral contraceptives [6]. Excessive weight gain was more prevalent among girls on DMPA. Twenty-five percent of females on DMPA gained more than 10% of their baseline body weight as compared with 7% of females on oral contraceptives after 1 year of use. In addition, adolescents who had gained more than 13.2 lbs in 1 year had a significantly greater baseline body mass index (BMI) compared with those with weight gain less than 13.2 lbs. Mangan and colleagues reviewed 239 adolescents (age: 19 years and younger) on DMPA or oral contraceptives and also found that overweight at time of DMPA initiation increased risk of weight gain [5]. Overweight adolescent females on DMPA gained significantly ($P < .05$) more weight at 1 year than overweight females on oral contraceptives (OCs), non-overweight females on DMPA, and nonoverweight females on OCs (13.6 lbs, 7.4 lbs, 6.9 lbs, 3.2 lbs, respectively).

Lastly, racial differences in DMPA-associated weight gain were identified by Polaneczky and colleagues [17]. Adolescent females (n = 159, mean age: 17.7 years) who had initiated DMPA were reviewed. At 11.1 months of use, mean weight gain for black subjects was 7.4 lbs as compared with 2.3 lbs for Hispanic subjects and 2.9 lbs for white subjects ($P < .02$).

Findings from prospective studies of adolescents on DMPA parallel those of retrospective studies. At 11 and 17 months of use, Matson and colleagues found significant weight gain among 53 African American adolescents (mean age: 16.5 years) on DMPA (6.0 kg and 9.0 kg, respectively) [20]. Again, no comparison group off DMPA was followed. Harel and colleagues conducted two studies examining the weight effects of DMPA use in adolescents [16,21]. Among a sample of 78 adolescents (age: 12 to 20 years), early second DMPA injection predisposed to greater weight gain as compared with the traditional 3-month dosing interval [21]. Whereas OC use before DMPA use was not associated with subsequent DMPA-related weight gain. In 35 adolescents (age: 13.5 to 21 years) who discontinued DMPA, significant weight gain ($P = .0005$)

Table 1
Studies evaluating weight changes in female adolescents on depot medroxyprogesterone acetate

Source (year)	Study design	Mean weight gain	Comments
Moore (1995) [18]	N = 150 Retrospective chart review, females aged 15–30 yrs on DMPA, OC or implants	At 1 year: DMPA: +0.1 lbs OC: −2.0 lbs Implants: −1.8 lbs	No significant wt gain in either group Race/ethnicity not reported
Harel (1995) [21]	N = 78 Prospective study, convenient sample of adolescents Group 1: received early second DMPA injection Group 2: DMPA at normal interval Group 3: went from OC to DMPA	At 3 months: Group 1: BMI + 0.99 kg/m^2 Group 2: BMI + 0.40 kg/m^2 Group 3: BMI + 0.38 kg/m^2	Early second DMPA injection predisposed to greater wt gain
Harel (1996) [16]	N = 35 Adolescents who discontinued DMPA	At discontinuation: BMI + 1.1 kg/m^2 (mean duration of use 9.2 months)	Significant wt gain that persisted for 6 months after discontinuation
Matson (1997) [20]	N = 53 Prospective study, African-American adolescents initiating DMPA	At 11 months: +6.0 kg At 17 months: +9.0 kg	Significant wt gain No concurrent control group
Polaneczky (1998) [17]	N = 159 Chart review and phone interview, adolescents who initiated DMPA	At 11.1 months: African-American subjects: +7.4 lbs Hispanic subjects: +2.3 lbs White subjects: −2.9 lbs	Racial differences in wt gain
Risser (1999) [6]	N = 130 Retrospective chart review, adolescents on DMPA or OC	Percentage gaining >10% baseline wt: DMPA: 25% OC: 7%	Disproportionate number on DMPA gained >10% of baseline wt

Study	Design	Results	Comments
Templeman (2000) [19]	N = 133 Retrospective chart review, adolescents Group 1: DMPA injections every 3 months Group 2: DMPA injections monthly × 3 then every 3 months	Group 1: 3 months: +2.7 lbs 6 months: +6.4 lbs 12 months: +9.8 lbs Group 2: 3 months: +0.9 lbs 6 months: +4.6 lbs 12 months: +7.7 lb	Significant wt gain in both groups
Mangan (2002) [5]	N = 239 Retrospective chart review, adolescents using OC or DMPA for 1 y	At 1 y: DMPA: +8.9 lbs OC: +4.8 lbs	Overweight at the initiation of DMPA was a risk factor for wt gain
Bonny (2004) [9]	N = 43 Longitudinal study, adolescents initiating DMPA	At 6 months: African-American subjects: +2.9 kg White subjects: +0.9 kg	Racial differences in wt gain Large adipose gains
Bonny (2004) [7,8]	N = 450 Prospective study, adolescents initiating DMPA, OC, or controls	At 18 months: Nonobese DMPA: +4.0 kg Nonobese OC: +2.8 kg Nonobese control: +3.5 kg Obese DMPA: +9.5 kg Obese OC: +0.2 kg Obese Control: +3.1 kg	Obese at time of DMPA initiation risk factor for wt gain

seen at time of DMPA discontinuation persisted for up to 6 months after stopping the method [16].

Bonny and colleagues prospectively followed 43 adolescents (age: 12 to 21 years) who initiated DMPA [9]. Similar to Polaneczky and colleagues [17], Bonny found racial differences in DMPA-associated weight gain. Black and white subjects did not differ in baseline body weight. At 6 months, black subjects experienced a 4.2% increase in weight from baseline ($P = .003$) as compared with a 1.2% increase ($P = .32$) among white subjects. This study also examined adiposity and weight gains and found even more significant results. At 6 months, black subjects experienced a 12.5% increase in body fat from baseline ($P < .001$) as compared with a 1.2% increase ($P = .54$) among white subjects. Eating behaviors, including appetite, were measured by these investigators and did not predict weight or adipose increases.

The largest controlled, prospective study to date, conducted by Bonny and colleagues, followed 450 adolescents (age: 12 to 18 years) initiating DMPA, OC, or no hormonal contraceptive method [7,8]. As in Mangan's study [5], this study found a significant ($P < .001$) interaction between baseline obesity status and contraceptive weight gain. DMPA use was associated significantly with increased rates of weight gain in obese subjects, whereas OC use was not. Over 18 months, obese adolescents on DMPA gained an average of 9.5 kg and experienced a mean BMI increase of 3.0 units. In contrast, mean weight gain among obese females on OC (0.2 kg) and obese females on no contraceptive (3.1 kg) was significantly ($P = .001$) lower. Furthermore, weight gain among obese females on DMPA was significantly ($P < .001$) higher than that seen in nonobese females on DMPA, OC or no method. Contraceptive method did not predict weight gain for nonobese individuals, and no effect of race or ethnicity on contraceptive weight gain was found in this study.

In summary, most studies evaluating weight gain in adolescents on DMPA suggest some effect; yet predictors and mechanisms of weight gain have remained relatively unexplored. Patients who are overweight at time of DMPA initiation appear to be at greatest risk. Weight gain is paralleled by significant increases in body fat, and eating behaviors do not appear to modulate the weight effect.

Depot medroxyprogesterone acetate and bone

High rates of bone acquisition normally occur during the early part of adolescence, with peak bone mineral accrual taking place at 12.5 plus or minus 0.9 years for girls [22]. Twenty-six percent of adult total bone mineral is accumulated around this peak accretion time [23,24]. Eighty percent to 90% of bone mineral content (BMC) has been achieved, and most epiphyses are closed by 16 years of age [25–29]. A period of consolidation then takes place after the cessation of linear growth, with 99% of peak BMC reached by 26 years of age in women. Thus adolescence through young adulthood is the critical time for bone mass accumulation.

Bone mass accumulation during adolescence and young adulthood is dependent on a number of endocrine factors. Increases in both growth hormone and sex steroid levels have positive effects on BMD [30,31]. In females, estrogen is a key determinant of BMD, with significant associations reported between gynecologic age (a measure of pubertal development) and BMD ($P < .05$) [32]. Significant increases in spine and total body BMD with rising Tanner stages also have been demonstrated [33]. A major mechanism by which estrogen reduces bone resorption is through inhibition of osteoclast function.

Concern about DMPA suppression of estradiol, thereby negating the antiresorptive effects of estrogen on bone, prompted researchers to examine the effect of DMPA on bone mass. Numerous reports examining the relationship between DMPA and bone in adolescent and young adult woman have shown mixed results. Six studies (two cross-sectional design and four prospective) have examined bone mass in female adolescents on DMPA [32,34–38]. These studies are outlined in Table 2.

Scholes and colleagues [35] and Tharnprisarn and Taneepanichskul [36] employed cross-sectional analyses to evaluate the relationship between DMPA use and BMD in adolescents. Scholes reported on the duration of use of DMPA retrospectively and its potential effect on BMD in adolescent females (age: 14 to 18 years) from the Group Health Cooperative in Washington State [35]. Adolescents on DMPA (n = 81) were found to have lower BMD at the hip, spine, and whole body as compared with adolescents not using the method (n = 93). A statistical trend was found between duration of DMPA exposure and BMD. The differences, however, were not statistically significant. Subjects who had received eight or more DMPA injections had a mean spine BMD of 0.946 g/cm^2, while subjects with only one injection had a mean spine BMD of 0.988 g/cm^2 (p = .06). In comparison, subjects not using DMPA had a mean spine BMD of 0.994 g/cm^2.

Tharnprisarn and Taneepanichskul compared nondominant forearm BMD in adolescent and young Thai women (age: 15 to 30 years) on DMPA or oral contraceptives [36]. Mean duration of method use was 27.8 months (plus or minus 14.6 SD) and 24.1 months (plus or minus 14.0 SD) for DMPA and OC, respectively. There was no significant difference in BMD at the ultradistal forearm or distal forearm between the two groups. The researchers did not stratify subjects by age, however, and did not adjust for lifestyle covariates such as dietary intake or physical activity patterns.

Inherent limitations in cross-sectional analysis, including uncontrolled covariates, may account for the lack of significant findings in Scholes' and Tharnprisarn's analyses. In addition, both these studies included predominantly older adolescent females, a period when most bone mass has been accrued, and bone consolidation is occurring. In the Scholes' analysis, only 23 of the DMPA subjects were 14 to 16 years of age, while 58 were 17 to 18 years of age. Mean age of subjects on DMPA from the Tharnprisarn's study was 24.6 plus or minus 3.3 years with only three subjects in the 16- to 19-year-old age group.

Table 2
Studies evaluating bone mineral density in female adolescents on depot medroxyprogesterone acetate

Source (year)	Study design	Bone mineral density	Comments
Scholes (2004) [35]	N = 174 Cross-sectional analysis, females 14–18 yrs, on DMPA or not using method (control)	Mean spine BMD (g/cm^2) DMPA: 0.97 Control: 0.994 Mean hip BMD (g/cm^2) DMPA: 0.94 Control: 0.970	No significant differences between groups Duration of DMPA use 1–39 months
Tharnsprisarn (2002) [36]	N = 60 Cross-sectional analysis, Thai females aged 15–30 yrs, on DMPA or OC for at least 2 yrs	Mean BMD (g/cm^2) Distal forearm: DMPA: 0.403 OC: 0.423 Ultradistal forearm: DMPA: 0.571 OC: 0.566	No significant differences between groups Control group included OC users
Busen (2002) [34]	N = 6 Prospective study, females aged 15–19 yrs on DMPA	At Yr 1: % Δ Spine BMD: −3.52% % Δ Hip BMD: −3.31%	Significant BMD loss No control group
Cromer (1996) [32]	N = 32 Prospective study, females aged 12–21 yrs on DMPA or no hormonal method	% Δ Spine BMD Yr 1: DMPA: −1.5% Control: +2.9% Yr 2: DMPA: −3.1% Control: +9.5%	Significant differences between groups at yr 1 and yr 2
Lara-Torre (2004) [37]	N = 77 Prospective study, females aged 12–21 yrs, on DMPA or no hormonal method	% Δ Spine BMD Yr 1: DMPA: −1.59% Control: +2.45% Yr 2: DMPA: −1.85% Control: +5.89%	Significant differences between groups at yr 1 and yr 2
Cromer (2004) [38]	N = 136 Prospective study, females aged 12–18 yrs, on DMPA or no hormonal method	At 1 yr: % Δ Spine BMD DMPA: −1.4% Control: +3.8% % Δ Hip BMD DMPA: −2.2% Control: +2.3%	Significant differences in spine and hip BMD between groups at yr 1

In four prospective studies on DMPA use and BMD in adolescents, significant differences between subjects on DMPA and controls were reported [32,34,37,38]. In a small sample (n = 6), Busen and colleagues examined changes in BMD in adolescents on DMPA (age: 15 to 19 years) [34]. At 1 year of use, a mean loss of bone at the femoral neck of −3.31% ($P = .013$) and at the lumbar spine of

−3.52% ($P=.02$) were found. Similarly, Lara-Torre and colleagues studied adolescents and young adult women (n = 77; age: 12 to 21 years) for 24 months with bone measurements conducted at 6-month intervals [37]. A significant difference in spine BMD was observed at each time point between subjects on DMPA and controls. Over the course of the study, subjects on DMPA had a negative mean change in lumbar spine BMD, while controls experienced a positive mean change. Thus when compared with controls, subjects on DMPA had a mean percent change in lumbar spine BMD of −3.01% at 6 months ($P=.014$), −3.02% at 12 months ($P=.001$), −4.81% at 18 months ($P<.001$), and −6.81% at 24 months ($P=.01$).

Cromer and colleagues have completed two prospective studies on DMPA and BMD in adolescent females [32,38]. In a small study in Columbus, Ohio, Cromer followed lumbar spine BMD changes in adolescents (age: 12 to 21 years) over 2 years and observed a decrease of −3.12% in subjects on DMPA (n = 8) compared with an increase of 9.49% in control participants (n = 4) ($P<.0001$) [32]. In a larger prospective study conducted in Cleveland, Ohio, Cromer followed BMD changes in the femoral neck and lumbar spine of postmenarcheal girls (age: 12 to 18 years) on DMPA (n = 29) or no hormonal contraceptive method (n = 107) [38]. At 1 year, subjects on DMPA experienced a −2.2% mean change at the femoral neck compared with 2.3% mean change for the controls ($P<.005$) and a −1.4% change at the lumbar spine compared with 3.8% change for the controls ($P<.001$) (Figs. 1, 2).

As mentioned, the proposed mechanism for DMPA-associated bone loss is low levels of estrogen from suppression of the hypothalamic-pituitary-ovarian axis. Evidence in support of this mechanism can be found in two studies that documented, through randomized controlled clinical trials, improvement in BMD on DMPA with estrogen supplementation [39,40]. In addition, Rome and colleagues observed higher levels of bone specific alkaline phosphatase (BSAP), an important marker of bone formation, in subjects not on hormonal contraception (n = 152; age: 12 to 18 years) as compared with adolescents on DMPA (n = 53;

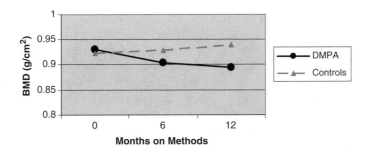

Fig. 1. Bone mineral density at the femoral neck in adolescent females on DMPA and controls. (*Data from* Cromer BA, Stager M, Bonny A, et al. Depot medroxyprogesterone acetate, oral contraceptives and bone mineral density in a cohort of adolescent girls. J Adolesc Health 2004;35: 434–41.)

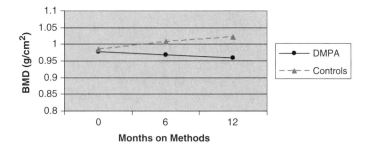

Fig. 2. Bone mineral density at the spine in adolescent females on DMPA and controls. (*Data from* Cromer BA, Stager M, Bonny A, et al. Depot medroxyprogesterone acetate, oral contraceptives and bone mineral density in a cohort of adolescent girls. J Adolesc Health 2004;35:434–41.)

age: 12 to 18 years) [41]. At 12 months of DMPA use, mean serum BSAP levels were 35.2 plus or minus 1.05 U/L versus 40.4 plus or minus 1.03 U/L ($P<.05$) for subjects on DMPA as compared with controls, respectively. Similarly, Ott and colleagues reported significant differences in bone resorption, measured by N-telopeptide (NTX), between subjects on DMPA and controls [42]. In a group of women (age: 18 to 39 years), mean NTX levels were 42.4 plus or minus 2.3 nmol/mmol creat and 35.4 plus or minus 2.9 nmol/mmol creat for DMPA and control subjects, respectively ($P<.01$).

In summary, evidence suggests that when compared with female adolescents not using hormonal contraception, adolescents on DMPA experience a relative loss of BMD. The speculative implication is that bone formation may be decreased and bone resorption increased in young women on DMPA as compared with untreated adolescents. Losses in BMD appear to increase with longer duration of use. Estrogen suppression appears to facilitate this response. It is unclear whether bone loss experienced on DMPA is reversible once the contraceptive method is stopped, particularly in the very young adolescent [43].

Implications for clinical practice

Optimal weight and bone health during adolescence depend on numerous factors, including hormonal, metabolic, genetic, and lifestyle influences. Maximizing modifiable lifestyle factors, such as diet and physical activity, for weight and bone health is essential for all adolescents on DMPA. For example, maximizing calcium intake during adolescence appears to influence the attainment of peak bone mass. In healthy children, calcium intake levels between 1200 and 1500 mg/d result in maximal net calcium balance. At lower calcium intakes, the skeleton may be deprived of needed calcium, and peak bone mass may not be reached [44–47].

Calcium intakes among female adolescents in the United States are substantially lower than 1200 to 1500 mg/d. Mean calcium intake from the 1999 to

2000 NHANES for females 12 to 19 years was 793 mg/d [48]. Nationally, from 1977 to 1978 to 1994 to 1996, milk intake among female adolescents decreased by 36% [49]. Supplementation trials with calcium support optimizing calcium intake to achieve peak bone mass [44,50–52]. In adult women (age: 30 to 45 years), one prospective study conducted by Merki-Feld and colleagues examined the effect of calcium intake and calcium supplementation on BMD while on DMPA [53]. In both women on DMPA and those off hormonal contraception, calcium intake was correlated significantly with trabecular bone mass ($P < .05$). Among women on DMPA, treatment with calcium and vitamin D supplementation during the second year of the study resulted in a lower annual trabecular bone loss as compared with the first year with no supplementation ($P < .08$).

Although there are no available data to indicate that optimizing dietary calcium to meet the Dietary Reference Intake (RDI) is supportive of bone health for adolescents on DMPA, it is apparent that calcium is important for adolescent bone mass accrual and is one clinical intervention that reasonably can be accomplished. In addition, several observational studies have detected inverse associations between calcium intake and body weight or body fat [54,55]. Thus, calcium supplementation of the adolescent on DMPA may benefit both body weight and bone health.

It is accepted that physical activity has a positive effect on weight, body composition, and bone mass. Moreover, the interaction between adequate dietary calcium and physical activity is important and should be emphasized [33,56,57] (ie, the combination of physical activity and calcium intake above 1000 mg/d appears to have a synergistic action on bone mass. Therefore, recommendations to increase dietary calcium intake should include emphasis on physical activity, especially weight-bearing exercise. These recommendations are particularly pertinent for those using DMPA.

Further management of the adolescent currently using or contemplating use of DMPA must include evaluation of the potential risk of unintended pregnancy. An estimated 10% of adolescent females will become pregnant between the ages of 15 and 19 [58]. The personal and social costs for adolescents with unplanned pregnancies are documented [59]. Parenthood impairs an adolescent's ability to acquire a complete education, deprives her of job opportunities, jeopardizes her ability to support herself and her family, and places her at increased risk for physical abuse [60,61]. The long-term consequences of adolescent pregnancy on weight or bone health are also not known.

Other forms of hormonal contraception, such as OCs, may be suitable alternatives to DMPA in some adolescents but are limited by poor compliance in others. Daily compliance with OCs in the adolescent age group is typically poor. Only 58% of adolescents report perfect compliance with oral contraceptives [11]. Epidemiological studies suggest typical use of OC among female adolescents has a failure rate of 5% to 18%, a rate 55% higher than that found in adults [62–64]. Hence, for some adolescents, contraceptive methods that require daily or weekly compliance may place them at increased risk of pregnancy. With this in mind, the authors propose the following guidelines for DMPA use and management in the adolescent.

With regards to weight concerns, DMPA should be used cautiously in obese females with BMI greater 30 kg/m^2 (cut point found to be associated with greatest risk of weight gain by Bonny and colleagues) [8]. In light of the recommended upper weight limit of 198 lbs for the transdermal patch, oral contraceptives containing 35 µg of ethinyl estradiol (EE) or higher are probably the best alternative in such patients. Recent evidence suggests that women of higher body weight (over 70.5 kg) are at greater risk for OC failure as compared with women of lower weight [65]. Risk of OC failure among overweight women appears to increase with decreasing dose of EE. For example, the relative risk (95% confidence interval) of OC failure for women weighing more than 70.5 kg, as compared with women weighing less, is 4.5 (1.4, 14.4) when on very low-dose OC (less than 35 µg EE), 2.6 (1.2, 5.9) when on low-dose OC (35 µg EE to no more than 50 µg) and 1.2 (0.4, 3.5) when on high-dose OC (50 µg or more of EE). Hence, a moderate or high-dose OC may be the best option in an obese adolescent. If the risk of unintended pregnancy is high, however, DMPA may still be the best alternative. For example, in a sexually active, obese adolescent with poor ability to comply with daily or weekly contraceptive regimens, DMPA-associated weight gain may be more acceptable than potential pregnancy.

With regards to bone concerns, one approach to clinical management of the patient on DMPA is to obtain bone densitometry after long-term DMPA use (eg, 2 years). Using published normative data tables of BMD values in adolescents [66–68], the clinician can check whether BMD values fall within the normal range. If BMD is low (eg, less than 10th percentile for chronologic age, weight, and race), the clinician may want to encourage the adolescent to switch to a hormonal contraceptive containing estrogen, such as oral contraceptives or the transdermal patch. Another alternative, particularly if densitometry is not a feasible option, is to limit use of DMPA to 2 years, especially in thin, white female adolescents with low dietary calcium intake or in those who have limited capacity for weight bearing activity, as these are common risk factors for osteopenia in the adolescent female.

Summary

In summary, DMPA remains an effective and easy-to-use contraceptive method for adolescents. Recent literature suggests that overweight teens may be at increased risk for weight gain while on this contraceptive method. Use of DMPA in the obese adolescent therefore should be done only after careful consideration of other contraceptive options and potential risk of unintended pregnancy.

In addition, new literature suggests decreases in BMD among adolescent females on DMPA, particularly with longer duration of use. The implications of this on adult bone health are unclear. Therefore, use of DMPA for more than 2 years should be done after careful consideration and possible assessment of BMD.

All adolescents who initiate DMPA should receive dietary assessment and counseling. Dietary assessment should include evaluation and recommendations for increased dietary calcium through food sources or supplementation. Individualized physical activity recommendations also should be developed for each female adolescent on DMPA.

References

[1] 3-month contraceptive injection approved. FDA Med Bull 1993;23(1):6–7.

[2] Nelson A. Merits of DMPA relative to other reversible contraceptive methods. J Reprod Med 2002;47:781–4.

[3] Piccinino LJ, Mosher WD. Trends in contraceptive use in the United States: 1982–1995. Fam Plann Perspect 1998;30:4–10.

[4] Institute AG. Teen pregnancy rates continue to decline. Contracept Technol Update 1999;20:81–2.

[5] Mangan SA, Larsen PG, Hudson S. Overweight teens at increased risk for weight gain while using depot medroxyprogesterone acetate. J Pediatr Adolesc Gynecol 2002;15:79–82.

[6] Risser WL, Gefter LR, Barratt MS, et al. Weight change in adolescents who used hormonal contraception. J Adolesc Health 1999;24:433–6.

[7] Bonny A, Camlin K, Harvey R, et al. Prospective analysis of weight changes in adolescent females initiating depot medroxyprogesterone acetate (DMPA), oral contraceptive pills (OC), or no hormonal contraceptive method. J Adolesc Health 2003;32:134.

[8] Bonny A, Ziegler J, Harvey R, et al. Relationship between baseline obesity status and subsequent weight gain in adolescent females initiating depot medroxyprogesterone acetate (DMPA), oral contraceptive pills (OC), or no hormonal contraceptive method. Pediatr Res 2004;55:9A.

[9] Bonny AE, Britto MT, Huang B, et al. Weight gain, adiposity, and eating behaviors among adolescent females on depot medroxyprogesterone acetate (DMPA). J Pediatr Adolesc Gynecol 2004;17:109–15.

[10] Food and Drug Administration. FDA Talk Paper. Black box warning added concerning long-term use of Depo-Provera contraceptive injection. Rockville (MD): Food and Drug Administration; 2004.

[11] Abma JC, Chandra A, Mosher WD, et al. Fertility, family planning, and women's health: new data from the 1995 National Survey of Family Growth. Vital Health Stat 1997;23:1–114.

[12] Jones EF. Teenage pregnancy in industrialized countries. New Haven (CT): Yale University Press; 1986.

[13] Rubinstein ML, Halpern-Felsher BL, Irwin CE. An evaluation of the use of the transdermal contraceptive patch in adolescents. J Adolesc Health 2004;34:395–401.

[14] Burkman RT, Miller L. Extended and continuous use of hormonal contraceptives. Dialogues Contracept 2004;8(4):1–3, 8.

[15] O'Dell CM, Forke CM, Polaneczky MM, et al. Depot medroxyprogesterone acetate or oral contraception in postpartum adolescents. Obstet Gynecol 1998;91:609–14.

[16] Harel Z, Biro FM, Kollar LM, et al. Adolescents' reasons for and experience after discontinuation of the long-acting contraceptives Depo-Provera and Norplant. J Adolesc Health 1996;19:118–23.

[17] Polaneczky M, Liblanc M. Long-term depot medroxyprogesterone acetate (Depo-Provera) use in inner-city adolescents. J Adolesc Health 1998;23:81–8.

[18] Moore LL, Valuck R, McDougall C, et al. A comparative study of one-year weight gain among users of medroxyprogesterone acetate, levonorgestrel implants, and oral contraceptives. Contraception 1995;52:215–9.

[19] Templeman C, Boyd H, Hertweck SP. Depomedroxyprogesterone acetate use and weight gain among adolescents. J Pediatr Adolesc Gynecol 2000;13:45–6.

[20] Matson SC, Henderson KA, McGrath GJ. Physical findings and symptoms of depot medroxyprogesterone acetate use in adolescent females. J Pediatr Adolesc Gynecol 1997;10:18–23.

[21] Harel Z, Biro FM, Kollar LM. Depo-Provera in adolescents: effects of early second injection or prior oral contraception. J Adolesc Health 1995;16(5):379–84.

[22] Bailey DA, Martin AD, McKay HA, et al. Calcium accretion in girls and boys during puberty: a longitudinal analysis. J Bone Miner Res 2000;15:2245–50.

[23] Bailey DA, McKay HA, Mirwald RL, et al. A six-year longitudinal study of the relationship of physical activity to bone mineral accrual in growing children: the university of Saskatchewan bone mineral accrual study. J Bone Miner Res 1999;14:1672–9.

[24] Slemenda CW, Reister TK, Hui SL, et al. Influences on skeletal mineralization in children and adolescents: evidence for varying effects of sexual maturation and physical activity. J Pediatr 1994;125:201–7.

[25] Henry YM, Fatayerji D, Eastell R. Attainment of peak bone mass at the lumbar spine, femoral neck and radius in men and women: relative contributions of bone size and volumetric bone mineral density. Osteoporos Int 2004;15:263–73.

[26] Matkovic V, Fontana D, Tominac C, et al. Factors that influence peak bone mass formation: a study of calcium balance and the inheritance of bone mass in adolescent females. Am J Clin Nutr 1990;52:878–88.

[27] Katzman DK, Bachrach LK, Carter DR, et al. Clinical and anthropometric correlates of bone mineral acquisition in healthy adolescent girls. J Clin Endocrinol Metab 1991;73:1332–9.

[28] Lu PW, Cowell CT, LLoyd-Jones SA, et al. Volumetric bone mineral density in normal subjects, aged 5–27 years. J Clin Endocrinol Metab 1996;81:1586–90.

[29] Bonjour JP, Theintz G, Buchs B, et al. Critical years and stages of puberty for spinal and femoral bone mass accumulation during adolescence. J Clin Endocrinol Metab 1991;73:555–63.

[30] Albertsson-Wikland K, Rosberg S, Karlberg J, et al. Analysis of 24-hour growth hormone profiles in healthy boys and girls of normal stature: relation to puberty. J Clin Endocrinol Metab 1994;78:1195–201.

[31] Frank GR. The role of estrogen in pubertal skeletal physiology: epiphyseal maturation and mineralization of the skeleton. Acta Paediatr 1995;84:627–30.

[32] Cromer BA, Blair JM, Mahan JD, et al. A prospective comparison of bone density in adolescent girls receiving depot medroxyprogesterone acetate (Depo-Provera), levonorgestrel (Norplant), or oral contraceptives. J Pediatr 1996;129:671–6.

[33] Boot AM, de Ridder MA, Pols HA, et al. Bone mineral density in children and adolescents: relation to puberty, calcium intake, and physical activity. J Clin Endocrinol Metab 1997;82:57–62.

[34] Busen NH, Britt RB, Rianon N. Bone mineral density in a cohort of adolescent women using depot medroxyprogesterone acetate for one to two years. J Adolesc Health 2003;32:257–9.

[35] Scholes D, LaCroix AZ, Ichikawa LE, et al. The association between depot medroxyprogesterone acetate contraception and bone mineral density in adolescent women. Contraception 2004; 69:99–104.

[36] Tharnprisarn W, Taneepanichskul S. Bone mineral density in adolescent and young Thai girls receiving oral contraceptives compared with depot medroxyprogesterone acetate: a cross-sectional study in young Thai women. Contraception 2002;66:101–3.

[37] Lara-Torre E, Edwards CP, Perlman S, et al. Bone mineral density in adolescent females using depot medroxyprogesterone acetate. J Pediatr Adolesc Gynecol 2004;17:17–21.

[38] Cromer BA, Stager M, Bonny A, et al. Depot medroxyprogesterone acetate, oral contraceptives and bone mineral density in a cohort of adolescent girls. J Adolesc Health 2004;35:434–41.

[39] Cromer B, Lazebnik R, Rome E, et al. A double-blind randomized controlled trial of estrogen supplementation in adolescent girls receiving depot medroxyprogesterone acetate for contraception. Am J Obstet Gynecol 2004;192(1):42–7.

[40] Cundy T, Ames R, Horne A, et al. A randomized controlled trial of estrogen replacement therapy in long-term users of depot medroxyprogesterone acetate. J Clin Endocrinol Metab 2003;88: 78–81.

[41] Rome E, Ziegler J, Secic M, et al. Bone biochemical markers in adolescent girls using either depot medroxyprogesterone acetate or an oral contraceptive. J Pediatr Adolesc Gynecol 2004;17: 373–7.

[42] Ott SM, Scholes D, LaCroix AZ, et al. Effects of contraceptive use on bone biochemical markers in young women. J Clin Endocrinol Metab 2001;86:179–85.

[43] Scholes D, LaCroix AZ, Ichikawa LE, et al. Injectable hormone contraception and bone density: results from a prospective study. Epidemiology 2002;13:581–7.

[44] Johnston Jr CC, Miller JZ, Slemenda CW, et al. Calcium supplementation and increases in bone mineral density in children. N Engl J Med 1992;327:82–7.

[45] Matkovic V. Calcium metabolism and calcium requirements during skeletal modeling and consolidation of bone mass. Am J Clin Nutr 1991;54:245S–60S.

[46] Abrams SA, Copeland KC, Gunn SK, et al. Calcium absorption, bone mass accumulation, and kinetics increase during early pubertal development in girls. J Clin Endocrinol Metab 2000; 85:1805–9.

[47] Jackman LA, Millane SS, Martin BR, et al. Calcium retention in relation to calcium intake and postmenarcheal age in adolescent females. Am J Clin Nutr 1997;66:327–33.

[48] Ervin RB, Wang CY, Wright JD, et al. Dietary intake of selected minerals for the United States population: 1999–2000. Advanced data from vital and health statistics; 341. Wrightsville (MD): National Center for Health Statistics; 2004.

[49] Bowman SA. Beverage choices of young females: changes and impact on nutrient intakes. J Am Diet Assoc 2002;102:1234–9.

[50] Andon MB, Lloyd T, Matkovic V. Supplementation trials with calcium citrate malate: evidence in favor of increasing the calcium RDA during childhood and adolescence. J Nutr 1994;124: 1412S–7S.

[51] Cadogan J, Eastell R, Jones N, et al. Milk intake and bone mineral acquisition in adolescent girls: randomized, controlled intervention trial. BMJ 1997;315:1255–60.

[52] Chan GM, Hoffman K, McMurry M. Effects of dairy products on bone and body composition in pubertal girls. J Pediatr 1995;126:551–6.

[53] Merki-Feld GS, Neff M, Keller PJ. A 2-year prospective study on the effects of depot medroxyprogesterone acetate on bone mass-response to estrogen and calcium therapy in individual users. Contraception 2003;67:79–86.

[54] Novotny R, Daida YG, Acharya S, et al. Dairy intake is associated with lower body fat and soda intake with greater weight in adolescent girls. J Nutr 2004;134:1905–9.

[55] Lin YC, Lyle RM, McCabe LD, et al. Dairy calcium is related to changes in body composition during a two-year exercise intervention in young women. J Am Coll Nutr 2000;19:754–60.

[56] Specker BL. Evidence for an interaction between calcium intake and physical activity on changes in bone mineral density. J Bone Miner Res 1996;11:1539–44.

[57] Rowlands AV, Ingledew DK, Powell SM, et al. Interactive effects of habitual physical activity and calcium intake on bone density in boys and girls. J Appl Physiol 2004;97:1203–8.

[58] Templeman CL, Cook V, Goldsmith LJ, et al. Postpartum contraceptive use among adolescent mothers. Obstet Gynecol 2000;95:770–6.

[59] Millstein S, Halpern-Felsher B. Adolescent sexuality. In: Blechman K, editor. Behavioral medicine and women: a comprehensive handbook. New York: Guilford Publications; 1998. p. 59–63.

[60] Dailard C. US policy can reduce cost barriers to contraception. Issues Brief (Alan Guttmacher Inst) 1999;2:1–4.

[61] Goodwin MM, Gazmararian JA, Johnson CH, et al. Pregnancy intendedness and physical abuse around the time of pregnancy: findings from the pregnancy risk assessment monitoring system, 1996–1997. PRAMS Working Group. Pregnancy Risk Assessment Monitoring System. Matern Child Health J 2000;4:85–92.

[62] Chacko MR, Kozinetz CA, Smith PB. Assessment of oral contraceptive pill continuation in young women. J Pediatr Adolesc Gynecol 1999;12:143–8.

[63] Brill SR, Rosenfeld WD. Contraception. Med Clin North Am 2000;84:907–25.

[64] Fu H, Darroch JE, Haas T, et al. Contraceptive failure rates: new estimates from the 1995 National Survey of Family Growth. Fam Plann Perspect 1999;31:56–63.

[65] Holt VL, Cushing-Haugen KL, Daling JR. Body weight and risk of oral contraceptive failure. Obstet Gynecol 2002;99:820–7.

[66] Horlick M, Wang J, Pierson Jr RN, et al. Prediction models for evaluation of total-body bone mass with dual-energy X-ray absorptiometry among children and adolescents. Pediatrics 2004;114:e337–45.

[67] Cromer BA, Binkovitz L, Ziegler J, et al. Reference values for bone mineral density in 12- to 18-year-old girls categorized by weight, race, and age. Pediatr Radiol 2004;34(10):787–92.

[68] Horlick M, Lappe JM, Gilsanz V, et al. The bone mineral density in childhood study (BMDCS): baseline results for 1554 health pediatric volunteers. J Bone Miner Res 2004;19:S14.

ELSEVIER
SAUNDERS

Adolesc Med 16 (2005) 585–602

ADOLESCENT
MEDICINE
CLINICS

Emergency Contraception

Lee Ann E. Conard, RPh, DO, MPH, Melanie A. Gold, DO*

*Division of Adolescent Medicine, University of Pittsburgh School of Medicine,
Children's Hospital of Pittsburgh, 3705 5th Avenue, Pittsburgh, PA 15213, USA*

In the United States, adolescent pregnancy rates have declined by 30% since 1991, with a record low of 43 births per 1000 women ages 15 to 19 in 2002 [1]. Although this is a positive trend, the United States still has a higher adolescent pregnancy rate than many other developed countries [2]. The use of contraceptives by adolescent women has been increasing, but adolescents as a group have higher rates of contraceptive failure compared with older women [3,4]. No contraceptive method is 100% effective, and even with perfect use and good technique, adolescents still may experience times of inadequate protection. Despite improvements in the accessibility and range of contraceptive options available, 8 of 10 adolescent pregnancies are unintended [5]. Timely use of emergency contraception (EC) could reduce the risk of pregnancy by as much as 89% to 99%, depending on the type used, and could prevent as many as 1.5 million unintended pregnancies each year [6].

Emergency contraception is recommended for any woman of reproductive age if she wants to lower her risk of becoming pregnant following unprotected or inadequately protected vaginal–penile intercourse. This includes failures of contraceptive methods such as a broken condom, dislodged diaphragm or cervical cap, forgotten combination oral contraceptive pills (COCs), a detached contraceptive patch, a removed vaginal contraceptive ring, late medroxyprogesterone acetate injection, or failed withdrawal (Table 1). Treatment also may be used in instances where no contraceptive method was used, such as sexual assault [6]. EC is increasing in use and has become a universal standard of care.

* Corresponding author.
E-mail address: magold@pitt.edu (M.A. Gold).

Table 1
Indications for using emergency contraception

Method	Reason for failure
Any time sex is unprotected	Nothing used, sexual assault
Condom	Breaks or slips
Combination oral contraceptive pills (COCs)	Started the pill within the past 7 days (but not during menses), and did not use a back-up method, or back-up method failed Missed two or more pills in a row during the first 3 weeks of any pack of pills More than 2 days late starting a new pack of pills after 7 days of placebo pills
Progestin only oral contraceptive pills (POPs)	Started the pill within the past 2 days (but not during menses), and did not use a back up or back up failed Missed one or more pills in any row of the pack More than one day late starting a new pack of pills
Transdermal patch	Started the patch within the past 7 days (but not during menses), and did not use a back up or back up failed Patch off >24 hours during patch-on weeks Left patch on for >9 days straight >2 days late putting patch back on after patch-off week
Vaginal ring	Started the ring within the past 7 days (but not during menses), and did not use a back-up method or back-up method failed Taken out for >3 hours during ring-in weeks Left in >5 weeks in a row >2 days late putting ring back in after ring-out week
Depot medroxyprogesterone acetate injection	Started within the past 14 days (but not within 5 days of menses) and did not use a back-up method or back-up method failed More than 13 weeks since last shot
Diaphragm or cervical cap	Slipped during intercourse Removed too early after intercourse (less than 6 hours)
Withdrawal	Did not wipe off tip of penis before vaginal penetration Ejaculation occurred while penis was inside the vagina
Spermicide	Put in more than an hour before intercourse Dose not repeated prior to subsequent episodes of intercourse Any time used without another back up (like a condom)

Products

There are three types of EC available in the United States: progestin only pills (POPs), COCs, and the copper-releasing intrauterine device (IUD). Outside of the United States, mifepristone also is used.

Two types of POPs are available in the United States. Plan B is a dedicated product that contains two tablets (0.75 mg each) of levonorgestrel. Ovrette usually is used for ongoing contraception; when used for EC, 20 tablets of Ovrette per dose (for a total of 40 tablets) would be required to obtain the appropriate dose of levonorgestrel.

Plan B should be initiated as soon as possible after unprotected intercourse. The Food and Drug Administration (FDA)-approved instructions for Plan B are to take one tablet as soon as possible after unprotected intercourse and to repeat the second single tablet dose in 12 hours. Recent data, however, show that the use of both tablets at the same time is as effective at pregnancy prevention as the two-dose regimen [7]. The FDA instructions state that the Plan B can be started up to 72 hours after unprotected intercourse, but recent data support its use up to 120 hours after coitus [8,9]. When using, Ovrette, the two doses (of 20 tablets each) should be taken 12 hours apart.

Plan B generally is priced at $25 to $35 per packet (two tablets) but may be more expensive or may not be available in some pharmacies. Ovrette (two packs) can cost up to $70 for the two packs that are needed to complete a full regimen of EC. In states where pharmacists can dispense EC, cost may be $50 to $55 including the counseling fee charged by the pharmacist [9].

Combined oral contraceptive pills also can be used for EC. The Yuzpe regimen, using combined estrogen–progestin pills, has been used since the 1970s. Table 2 shows products that can be used for EC. The FDA has only recognized POPs and COCs with levonorgestrel or norgestrel for use as EC. A recent study, however, found that COCs with norethindrone can be effective for EC when compared with the standard Yuzpe regimen [10,11]. Because of the estrogen content, nausea is common when COCs are used for EC, and an anti-emetic medication should be offered for pretreatment when COCs are used for EC. Anti-emetics should be given at least 30 to 60 minutes before the first COC dose; meclizine may be a particularly good choice because of its 24-hour duration of action as compared with shorter acting anti-emetics such as dimenhydrinate, trimethobenzamide, or promethazine. One cycle of COCs may vary. Price may be as high as $50 [6,9].

Preven, a dedicated Yuzpe regimen product, was approved for use as an EC in 1998. Preven was taken off the market in 2004, because Gynetics sold the rights to the medication to Barr Laboratories. Barr then discontinued the product, because the company felt Plan B was a superior product. Because of the estrogen content, nausea was common with Preven (as it is with all Yuzpe regimens of EC), and women for whom estrogen use is contraindicated are safer taking a progestin-only regimen of EC than a Yuzpe regimen [9].

The copper IUD has been used for EC since the late 1970s. It can be placed in the uterus within 5 days of unprotected intercourse. This method should be

Table 2
Oral contraceptive pills for emergency contraception

Brand	Number of pills per dose (repeated in 12 hours)	Total ethinyl estradiol per dose (in μg)	Progestin type	Total levonorgestrel per dose (in mg)
Plan B	1 white*	0	LNG	0.75
Ovrette	20 yellow	0	NG	0.75
Aviane	5 orange	100	LNG	0.50
Levlite	5 pink	100	LNG	0.50
Lessina	5 pink	100	LNG	0.50
Alesse	5 pink	100	LNG	0.50
Ovral	2 white	100	NG	0.50
Ogestrel	2 white	100	NG	0.50
Enpresse	4 orange	120	LNG	0.50
Triphasil	4 yellow	120	LNG	0.50
Tri-Levlen	4 yellow	120	LNG	0.50
Trivora	4 pink	120	LNG	0.50
Seasonale	4 pink	120	LNG	0.60
Portia	4 pink	120	LNG	0.60
Nordette	4 light orange	120	LNG	0.60
Levlen	4 light orange	120	LNG	0.60
Low-Ogestrel	4 white	120	NG	0.60
Lo/Ovral	4 white	120	NG	0.60
Levora	4 white	120	LNG	0.60
Cryselle	4 white	120	NG	0.60

Abbreviations: LNG, levonorgestrel; NG, norgestrel.
  * Both doses may be taken at the same time [7].
Adapted from Stewart F, Trussell J, Van Look PF. Emergency contraception. In: Hatcher RA, Trussell J, Stewart F, et al, editors. Contraceptive technology. New York: Ardent Media; 2004. p. 279–303.

considered particularly when a woman wants to continue the IUD as her ongoing contraceptive method. Women should be in stable, mutually monogamous relationships with a low-risk for sexually transmitted infections (STIs). Adolescent women may not meet these criteria. The levonorgestrel IUD should not be used postcoitally, as its efficacy as an EC has never been assessed. The copper IUD can be expensive (around $500), and it has traditionally not been recommended for adolescents as EC, because of increased risk for STIs [9].

Mifepristone is an antiprogestin that blocks progesterone by binding to the receptor. It stops or prevents ovulation and disrupts the luteal phase or endometrial development. Mifepristone may be given in a single 10 mg dose within 120 hours of unprotected intercourse. Efficacy has been found to be similar to that of Plan B. It has fewer adverse effects than the Yuzpe regimen, but it can cause a slight delay in the next menses. Mifepristone is not available for use as EC in the United States [6].

Efficacy

An early study compared the efficacy and adverse effects of the Yuzpe regimen to the two-dose levonorgestrel regimen [12]. Both medications were

Table 3
Failure rates: Yuzpe levonorgestrel

Timing when pills were taken after unprotected sex	Yuzpe	Levonorgestrel
≤24 hours	2.0%	0.4%
25–48 hours	4.1%	1.2%
49–72 hours	4.7%	2.7%
Overall	3.2%	1.1%

given in divided doses 12 hours apart and were initiated within 72 hours of unprotected intercourse. This study noted that the earlier the treatment was given, the more effective it was; however, the overall pregnancy rate with levonorgestrel was 1.1% compared with 3.2% in the Yuzpe group (Table 3) [12]. In addition, women who used levonorgestrel had significantly less nausea and vomiting compared with those taking the Yuzpe regimen.

A second study by Piaggio reviewed data from previous studies (several of which found no significant effect of timing of initiation of the Yuzpe regimen on efficacy) and found that both the Yuzpe and levonorgestrel regimens were more effective the earlier treatment was started. By delaying the first dose of EC for 12 hours, the odds of pregnancy increased by 50% [13].

The original Yuzpe regimen of COCs (in terms of dose and timing) was empirically based. Newer regimens, however, have been studied that include extending the treatment period from 72 to 120 hours after unprotected intercourse, using combination COCs with norethindrone instead of levonorgestrel or norgestrel, administering a single dose of the Yuzpe regimen, administering the total progestin-only regimen of levonorgestrel in a single dose, and using mifepristone [7,8,11].

Women in one study were given the Yuzpe regimen, and their use was analyzed by timing of initiation: receiving it within 72 hours (N = 131) or between 72 and 120 hours (N = 169). The observed pregnancy rate was 1.1% (95% confidence intervals (CIs) 0 to 6.2 and 0.5.9) for both groups, and the effectiveness was 87% (95% CI 44.4% to 100% and 46.7% to 100%) for both groups. The Chi square tests were significant for both groups ($P < .5$), and observed pregnancy rates were lower than expected pregnancy rates without treatment [14].

A randomized controlled trial was conducted with 2041 women requesting EC within 72 hours of unprotected intercourse to assess the efficacy and side effects of three regimens of EC: the standard two-dose Yuzpe regimen, a single, first-dose Yuzpe regimen, and a Yuzpe variant using norethindrone instead of levonorgestrel [11]. Perfect-use failure rates were low for all three regimens (2.0%, 2.9%, and 2.7% respectively), and differences in failure rates by method were not statistically significant (Table 4) [11]. Adverse effects were similar for the standard Yuzpe regimen, and the Yuzpe variation with norethindrone, but the women in the group with one dose of Yuzpe experienced significantly less vomiting. Another finding from this study was that earlier time of initiation of EC was not associated with higher efficacy as was demonstrated in prior EC studies [11].

Table 4
Failure rates (% pregnant) with use of three Yuzpe regimens

	Perfect use	Typical use
Yuzpe standard (n = 585)	2.1%	2.5%
Yuzpe with norethindrone as the progestin component (n = 545)	2.8%	2.8%
Yuzpe (single dose only) (n = 542)	2.8%	3.4%

A second branch of the same study assessed the impact of extending the 72-hour time limit for EC to 120 hours. One hundred and eleven women enrolled in the study presented between 72 and 120 hours after unprotected intercourse; they were offered the standard Yuzpe regimen of EC when they refused IUD insertion. Perfect use (1.9%) and typical use (3.6%) failure rates were low and did not differ statistically from failure rates for the standard Yuzpe regimen when it was taken within the 72 hour time limit [8]. This result is consistent with the findings of others that levonorgestrel and mifepristone EC regimens are effective when the time limit is extended to 120 hours after unprotected intercourse [7]. This earlier study compared the efficacy of a single 10 mg dose of mifepristone, two 0.75 mg doses of levonorgestrel (standard) given 12 hours apart, and a single 1.5 mg dose of levonorgestrel given within 120 hours of unprotected intercourse. There were no significant differences between the groups in terms of pregnancy rates. Adverse effects were mild and did not differ significantly between groups [7].

Another study in China examined the effectiveness of a 10 mg dose of mifepristone for EC when given within 120 hours of unprotected intercourse. The pregnancy rate was 1.4%, with an estimated 82% of pregnancies prevented. Only 9% of the women taking mifepristone experienced nausea and vomiting [15]. A meta-analysis of mifepristone studies suggested a small dose effect on efficacy for doses less than 50 mg, and the pregnancy rate increased by 1.6 times when the dose was 10 mg instead of 25 mg. The authors noted, however, that one extra pregnancy for every 146 women requesting EC may be a low cost compared with the benefit of more women having access to mifepristone EC, because the monetary cost of a lower dosage may be less [16].

As research has progressed, more information has become available to estimate the efficacy of EC. Trussell and colleagues used new estimates of conception probabilities for estimating absolute levels of efficacy with data from a World Health Organization (WHO) clinical trial and from the Population Council trial [7,11,17]. Women in the WHO study were given levonorgestrel or the standard Yuzpe regimen. Women in the Population Council trial were given the standard Yuzpe regimen, only the first dose of the Yuzpe regimen, or a modified Yuzpe regimen with norethindrone substituted for levonorgestrel. With new methods of estimation, the effectiveness rate of EC dropped from 59.3% in the Population Council trial to 53.0% and from 62.5% to 46.8% in the WHO trial. The study also noted that cost-effectiveness was overestimated [17]. Raymond and colleagues determined that the levonorgestrel regimen prevented at least 49%

of pregnancies that might have been expected with the Yuzpe regimen. Therefore the minimum effectiveness of levonorgestrel at preventing pregnancy is 49% (95% CI 17% to 69%) assuming the Yuzpe method is ineffective (using it as a placebo). Because it is known that the Yuzpe method has some efficacy, the effectiveness of levonorgestrel is likely higher than the 49% estimate [18].

The copper-releasing IUD is the most effective method of EC available. The failure rate is less than 1%, or about six pregnancies per 1000 devices inserted [6].

Mechanism of action

The exact mechanism of action for oral EC regimens is not known. Because women who do not understand the mechanism of action of EC or have misconceptions about how it works are less likely to use it, one of the most important efforts in recent research is to increase understanding about how EC works to prevent pregnancy [19]. One of the main concerns is whether these EC regimens interfere with implantation of a fertilized egg, because some women and health care providers are uncomfortable with post-fertilization methods of contraception [20].

When taken before ovulation, oral EC regimens work primarily by disrupting normal follicular development and maturation so that ovulation does not occur or is delayed [6]. There also may be a deficient luteal phase and thickened cervical mucous [6]. When taken after ovulation, fertilization may have already taken place, and EC may work by altering the endometrial lining so implantation is less likely to occur [6]. Other proposed but less supported mechanisms of action include impaired sperm function or altered transport of sperm, egg, or blastocyst [6].

One recent study evaluating the effects of levonorgestrel and mifepristone on ovulation found that the luteinizing hormone (LH) peak was suppressed or delayed and that follicle rupture was inhibited [21]. The impact of levonorgestrel on ovulation, fertilization, and implantation in rats was assessed in another study. High-dose, postcoital levonorgestrel had no effect on implantation. Levonorgestrel, when given postcoitally to Cebus monkeys, had no effect on the pregnancy rate and had no postfertilization effect [20,22].

It is known that the Yuzpe regimen can suppress the LH peak partially or totally, and if given at the appropriate time, can inhibit follicle rupture [20]. Eight studies of women who used the Yuzpe regimen were assessed and compared with estimates of conception probabilities by cycle day of intercourse among women not using contraception. When women took EC following an episode of intercourse that occurred earlier in the cycle (on or before the day before ovulation), estimated effectiveness was 81%, but effectiveness was significantly lower (17%) for intercourse that occurred later in the cycle. These data support delaying ovulation as the primary mechanism of action of oral forms of EC and do not support the hypothesis that inhibition of implantation of a fertilized egg is a primary mechanism of action of EC [23].

Mifepristone acts as an antiprogestin by binding to progesterone receptors. In addition to the action described in the follicular phase, it also slows endometrial maturation in the luteal phase [21]. The copper-containing IUD may have some of the same mechanisms of action as oral EC, but because it has significantly higher efficacy than oral EC, it is felt that the copper IUD may work on tubal cilial motility to disrupt transport, and it also may work after fertilization by interfering with implantation [24]. The mechanism of action is more likely caused by a sterile inflammatory response in the uterus that makes fertilization unlikely, because the inflammatory response is toxic to sperm and possibly ova [25].

Adverse effects and complications

Adverse effects

Adverse effects from POPs are minor and less than those that occur with COCs. A recent study evaluated the tolerability of levonorgestrel EC (given in two doses) in adolescent women (N = 52) and found that the most reported adverse effects in the first week were headache (50%), fatigue (21%), nausea (38%), and dizziness (27%). The symptoms were reassessed in the second week after the medication was taken (when it would no longer be in the body), and 33% reported headache; 19% reported fatigue; 17% reported lower abdominal pain, and 13% reported nausea. Symptoms that were significantly higher in the first week were nausea ($P = .001$), fatigue ($P = .002$), headache ($P = .004$), and diarrhea ($P = .004$). Menses returned within 7 days of the anticipated date in 62.5% of participants [26].

Adverse effects from COCs used for EC include usual symptoms from the estrogen component, such as nausea, vomiting, breast tenderness, and headache. Nausea has been reported in 50% of women using the Yuzpe regimen, with vomiting occurring in 20%, while these symptoms are half as common in women taking progestin only EC (23% and 6% respectively) [12]. One large trial (N = 1973) of women ages 16 to 45 using the standard two-dose Yuzpe regimen found that 54% reported nausea; 16% reported vomiting; 12% reported headache; 8% reported fatigue; 6% reported dizziness, and 4% reported stomachache [11]. Other common adverse effects include breast tenderness and moodiness [9].

Another adverse effect after taking EC (POPs or COCs) can be vaginal spotting. One brief study reported a subset of data from a larger study of EC regimens on bleeding patterns following EC use. Among women who used any of the three regimens (the standard two-dose Yuzpe regimen, only the first dose of the Yuzpe regimen, or a variant of the Yuzpe regimen with norethindrone instead of levonorgestrel), 10% had spotting at some time before the next menses, and this usually lasted 1 to 2 days. There was no difference in spotting rates between women who became pregnant following EC use and those who did not. Women who took EC in the first half of the menstrual cycle (before day 12) were more likely to have their next period earlier than expected (by greater than 3 days) [27].

Adverse effects of mifepristone were reported for three randomized trials of the 10 mg dose. The percentage of women with nausea ranged from 0% to 19.4%; vomiting ranged from 0% to 4.3%, and lower abdominal pain ranged from 4.3% to 19.1%. The percentage of women with menstrual delay more than 7 days after expected date ranged from 4.3% to 25.8% [28]. Adverse effects from the copper-releasing IUD include pain, cramping with menses, bleeding, and infection. The IUD can increase menstrual blood loss by 50% during the first cycles after insertion [6,9,25].

Contraindications to use of POPs are pregnancy and allergy to a component of the product. FDA labeling of Plan B includes undiagnosed abnormal genital bleeding as a third contraindication [6,9]. For COCs, there are more contraindications because of the estrogen in the medication. Current pregnancy, allergy, and acute current migraine with neurologic deficits are absolute contraindications to prescribing the Yuzpe regimen. Although personal history of deep vein thrombosis (DVT) and pulmonary embolism (PE) is an absolute contraindication for ongoing contraception with a COC, it is not a contraindication for prescribing the Yuzpe regimen. In these clinical scenarios, however, it would be prudent to choose a progestin only EC regimen and reserve prescribing the Yuzpe regimen only if no progestin only EC regimen is available. The risk of clot for a patient with personal history of DVT or PE remains higher for pregnancy than for a single course of the Yuzpe regimen [6,9].

Complications

With 4 million doses of dedicated COC pills given for EC in the United Kingdom, three cases of DVT and three cases of cerebrovascular disorder have been reported, with none of these cases having clear links to the medication [29]. As EC has become more available, use has increased, and new adverse events have been reported. Cases of ectopic pregnancy previously had been reported in association with the Yuzpe regimen, but more recently, cases of ectopic pregnancy following the use of levonorgestrel EC have been reported also [30]. Gainer and colleagues reported that in 4 years of postmarketing surveillance in the European Union, 4.4 million units of levonorgestrel product were sold, and eight ectopic pregnancies were reported. They noted that in real-world use, if EC use resulted in a 3% failure rate, then 70,000 pregnancies and a minimum of 700 ectopic pregnancies should have been reported [31]. These data do not support an increased risk of ectopic pregnancy following the use of levonorgestrel EC. Two limitations of these studies are that it is unknown how many women actually took EC, and that the number of ectopic pregnancies may have been under-reported. At this time, it is unlikely that levonorgestrel EC increases the risk of ectopic pregnancy, because it is very effective at preventing pregnancy, and the ectopic rate may be lower than it would be in among women who did not use EC. Prior ectopic pregnancy is not a contraindication to

EC use. It may be prudent to confirm EC was effective, however, by checking a pregnancy test 2 weeks after EC is taken among women who have a history of ectopic pregnancy.

Another recent finding is that a woman's risk for pregnancy is particularly high if she has unprotected intercourse soon after taking EC. In a Chinese study, those women who took 10 mg of mifepristone and had unprotected sex after taking EC had 12 times the risk for pregnancy compared with women who used contraception or did not have intercourse after taking EC [15]. A second study showed that the relative risk of pregnancy was 28 times higher in women who had unprotected intercourse between treatment with mifepristone and onset of menses compared with women who reported no intercourse [28]. These studies demonstrate the importance of counseling women who take EC about the very rapid return of fertility and the need for interim abstinence or immediate initiation of contraception.

Complications of IUD use include uterine perforation (less than 1 in 1000 insertions) and expulsion (1 to 7 per 100 insertions in the first year) [25]. If a woman becomes pregnant with the copper IUD in place, it is not teratogenic to the fetus and may be removed in the first trimester. If the IUD is left in place, the woman may be at increased risk for preterm labor and spontaneous abortion [9].

Starting or restarting a method of contraception after use of emergency contraception

Because one of the primary ways that EC works to prevent pregnancy is by delaying ovulation, it is possible to be at risk for pregnancy in the first few days after completing EC treatment. Abstinence is recommended for 2 weeks after EC use. If an adolescent has a regular method of contraception, it should be restarted immediately (Table 5) [6]. If the adolescent wishes to begin a method of contraception or change methods, the health care provider can review the options

Table 5
Contraceptive instructions after use of emergency contraception

Method	When to use	Back-up method or abstinence
Was using COCs, POPs, transdermal patch or vaginal ring prior to EC use or wishes to initiate use	Restart the method the same day or the next day	1–2 weeks, pregnancy test in 2 weeks
Late for depot medroxyprogesterone acetate injection	2 weeks after use of EC, with a negative pregnancy test	Abstinence for 2 weeks after use of EC, then pregnancy test, then back-up method for 2 weeks after shot
Not restarting a hormonal method	None	Menstrual period should occur in the next 3 weeks, if not, a pregnancy test should be done

with her and counsel her to start the method as soon as possible. If the menstrual period does not return in 3 weeks, or if the adolescent is worried about pregnancy, a pregnancy test should be done at least 2 weeks after the last episode of unprotected intercourse.

Barrier methods, such as condoms, spermicides, and diaphragms can be used immediately. If combination or progestin only oral contraceptive pills were missed, they can be restarted the day after EC was taken. There is no need to catch up on missed pills. If restarting oral contraceptives, the patient can initiate a new package, either with the next menstrual cycle, or preferably taking one tablet every day starting the day after taking EC. If she used her regular COCs for EC, the adolescent can resume taking one pill per day from the same package, skip the placebo pills at the end of the pack, and go straight to the next package of pills. A backup method of contraception, such as a condom, should be used for 7 days. For those adolescents taking POPs, a new package should be started with the next menstrual cycle or preferably taking one tablet per day starting the day after taking EC. A back-up method should be used for 2 days. For the vaginal ring or patch, the method should be started the day after taking EC, or within 5 days of starting the next menstrual period. A back-up method should be used for the first 7 days when the patch or ring is restarted any time other than during menses. If she was getting depot medroxyprogesterone acetate injection shots but was late, and the patient just took EC, it is safest to advise the adolescent to not have intercourse for 2 weeks and then have a pregnancy test 2 weeks after taking EC. If her pregnancy test is negative, she can get another shot but should be counseled that she will not be protected from pregnancy for 14 days after restarting the shot [6,9]. All adolescents should be encouraged to consider testing for sexually transmitted diseases 14 days after the episode of unprotected intercourse.

Impact on sexual and contracepting behaviors

Some clinicians and women fear that providing EC may lead women to have more unprotected intercourse and may decrease the use of regular methods of contraception [32]. Eight studies demonstrate that these concerns are unfounded. An early study from the United Kingdom evaluated advance provision of EC and behavior in women ages 16 to 44 years. Forty-seven percent (N = 180) of the advance provision group used EC at least once compared with 27% (N = 87) of women in the control group who needed a study visit to get EC. Of those in the advance provision group, 98% of those who took EC used it correctly. There were 18 pregnancies in the advance provision group, compared with 25 pregnancies in the control group. The women in the advance provision group were not more likely to use EC repeatedly, and they used other methods of contraception at the same rate as women in the control group [33].

A study in Ghana of spermicide users compared behaviors of adult women who were given an advance supply of EC with those who had to return to clinic to receive EC. Women in both the advance supply and the on-demand groups used EC after 78% to 100% of unprotected coital acts, but EC was used sooner by the advance group (within 1 day of intercourse) than the on-demand group (within 2 to 3 days of intercourse). The two groups did not differ in frequency of unprotected intercourse [34].

In India, women (N = 411, nine subjects younger than 20 years) who used condoms for birth control were given information about EC (N = 198) or information and an advance supply of EC (N = 213). Women in both groups reported almost equal amounts of unprotected intercourse (0.012 acts per month for the advance supply group versus 0.016 acts per month for the information-only group). Of the advance-supply group, 98% said that having EC available did not cause them to lower their condom use [35].

In another study, postpartum women (mean age 25.6 years, with 18% of subjects younger than 20 years) were randomized to receive either an advance supply of EC or information on how to access EC on an as-needed basis. Women provided with advance EC were four times more likely to use EC over the course of the 1-year follow-up (17% versus 4%, RR 4.0, 95% CI 1.8, 9.0). Women in the advance provision group were not more likely to change to a less effective method of birth control (30% versus 33%, relative risk [RR] 0.92, 95% CI 0.63, 1.3) or to report using contraception less consistently (18% versus 25%, RR 0.74, 95% CI 0.45, 1.2). Close to half of the women in each group reported at least one episode of unprotected intercourse. For women who reported unprotected intercourse, those with a supply of EC were six times as likely to have used it compared with those in the control group (25% versus 4%, RR 5.8, 95% CI 2.1, 16.4) [36].

A recent advance provision study of women (N = 1030) (ages 18 to 45 years) in China found that in the advance supply group, younger women (younger than 26 years of age) were more likely to use a dose of EC than older women (47% versus 23%, P < .001). Women with an advance supply of EC used it almost three times more often than women who had to attend a clinic to receive EC (P < .001). During the study, the pattern of condom use was unchanged in both groups, and women in both groups stated that they were using contraception more consistently during the study. The pregnancy rate was similar in both groups [37].

Three studies assessed the impact of providing advance EC on adolescent behavior. One advance provision study of young women (ages 16 to 24 years) evaluated EC use, frequency of unprotected intercourse, and patterns of contraceptive use 4 months after enrollment. Women in the advance provision group were almost three times as likely as those in the control group to report using EC during the 4-month study (20% versus 7%, P = .006). Almost half of the women (46%) reporting using the same contraceptive method at enrollment and at follow-up. The proportion of young women who reported "never had unprotected sex" increased from enrollment to follow-up (33% versus 56%). At follow-up, however, women in the control group were more likely to report consistent oral contraceptive use than women in the advance supply group (58% versus 32%, P = .03) [38].

In a second advance provision study with adolescents, ages 15 to 20 years, there were no differences between advance EC and control groups in reported unprotected intercourse within the past month or at last intercourse at 1- and 6-month follow-up interviews. Additionally, there were no significant differences by group in hormonal contraception use reported at either past month or at last intercourse at the 1- or 6-month follow-up interviews. There was higher past month condom use reported among the advance provision group at the 6-month follow-up (77% versus 62%, $P = .02$). At the 1-month follow-up, the advance group reported nearly twice as much EC use as the control group (15% versus 8%, $P = .05$), and the advance provision group used EC sooner after unprotected intercourse (mean 11.4 hours versus 21.8 hours, $P = .005$) compared with the control group [39].

In the most recent advance provision study published in 2005, investigators assessed the sexual and contraceptive behaviors of young women, ages 15 to 24 years, who were randomized to one of three EC access groups: advance provision (with three packs of EC), pharmacy access, or clinic access (control group). Those in the advance provision group were almost twice as likely to use EC as those in the clinic access group at the 6-month follow-up (37.4% versus 21%, $P<.001$). The pharmacy access group, however, was not more likely to use EC compared with the clinic access group (24.4% versus 21.0%, $P = .25$). The advance provision group did not have significantly higher frequency of unprotected intercourse compared with the clinic access group (39.8% versus 40.1%, $P = .46$). No other differences in contraceptive or condom use or other sexual behaviors by group were found. At the 6-month follow-up, 8% of young women in the study had become pregnant, and 12% had acquired an STI. There were no reductions in pregnancies or increases in STIs by group (advance provision, pharmacy access, or clinic access) [40].

Access to and advance provision of emergency contraception

Practitioners routinely should provide information and counseling about EC to both female and male patients, at routine visits and at visits for contraceptive care. This information may be particularly helpful to sexually inexperienced adolescents, because they may be less likely to plan for unexpected sexual activity. Counseling should take into account the adolescent's age, developmental level, sexual orientation, and sexual history. During clinical encounters, sexually active females should be asked about the timing of the last vaginal intercourse, method of contraception, and whether there was any method failure. If the adolescent reports she had an episode of unprotected intercourse within the past 120 hours, EC should be offered (either as a prescription or better yet dispensing the medication in the office). All female adolescents receiving health care related to sexual assault should be counseled about EC, and the medication should be offered, if desired [41,42].

Office visits, pregnancy testing, pelvic examinations, Pap smears, or tests for STIs before prescribing or dispensing EC can pose significant barriers to timely access and rarely are indicated. Confidentiality that is required for other reproductive health care should be maintained for EC. Providers should consider offering an advance prescription or advance course of EC for adolescents to have on hand in the event of a future episode of unprotected intercourse or contraceptive failure. When a prescription is given, clinicians are encouraged to provide the adolescent with a list of local pharmacies known to carry EC. Because of higher efficacy and fewer adverse effects, Plan B should be the EC of choice (given as two tablets in a single dose); prescribers should only resort to a Yuzpe regimen using COCs when Plan B is unavailable in a timely manner [9,41,42].

Pharmacists can help increase access to EC, because they often advise patients, and may decide which medications to keep in stock; however, pharmacists may not feel comfortable with adolescent issues [43]. In one study, pharmacists in Pennsylvania were contacted by mystery shoppers and asked about EC. Among those surveyed, 49% of pharmacists could identify EC as birth control pills or hormones taken in high doses, and 33% knew the correct time interval for use, while 13% incorrectly said that EC causes an abortion. Most pharmacists (78%) correctly told the patient to contact her family physician or gynecologist to get a prescription for EC, but only 35% of pharmacists reported they had the medication in stock and could dispense EC that same day. Most (79%) of those who reported they could not fill the prescription the same day said that they did not have the medication in stock; 6% said it was against store policy, and 7% said that it conflicted with their personal beliefs [44]. In New Mexico, women visited pharmacies (N=178 visits) and found that dedicated EC products were in stock at 11% of pharmacy visits. Fifty-three percent of the pharmacies could obtain EC within 24 hours. Reasons for not stocking EC included lack of perceived need (65%), corporate decision not to stock (6%), and local decision not to stock (7%) [45].

As pharmacists widen their scope of practice, many states are allowing expanded prescribing authority. As of 2002, at least 35 states allowed pharmacists to have collaborative practice agreements with physicians that may involve approving refills and initiating and changing certain medication regimens. As of Nov. 1, 2004, pharmacists in four states had collaborative practice agreements specifically for EC: Alaska, California, Hawaii, and Washington. Pharmacists in California, Maine, and New Mexico have independent prescribing authority for EC [46].

There is hope that Plan B might become an over-the-counter (OTC) medication in the United States. On April 21, 2003, an application was submitted to the FDA for OTC status. On Dec. 16, 2003, two FDA committees voted 23:4 in favor of Plan B going OTC. On May 6, 2004, however, the FDA rejected the application, because it claimed there was insufficient information about how younger adolescents would use EC OTC. Barr Laboratories submitted an application to the FDA July 22, 2004, for a unique and unprecedented dual prescribing status for Plan B, suggesting that Plan B be OTC for women ages 16 and older but remain a prescription-only product for girls 15 and younger. A response to that application is pending.

Using behavior change counseling to facilitate emergency contraception use

Behavior change counseling, an adaptation of motivational interviewing, is a patient-centered approach that can be used to help the health care provider assess an adolescent's level of knowledge about EC and can facilitate her appropriate use of this information to make an informed decision [47–49]. One way to talk to an adolescent about EC would be to ask the patient during a conversation about pregnancy prevention, "What would you do if your 'Plan A' (regular method of contraception) for pregnancy prevention failed"? For a patient who uses oral contraceptive pills and condoms, she can be asked, "What can you do to prevent pregnancy if you forget two or more pills and you use a condom as a back-up but it breaks"? If she is able to describe EC as her plan, the health care provider can affirm that it is wonderful that she knows what to do and can continue to ask questions about what she knows about EC until misinformation is uncovered. Examples of questions can include: "What is it? Where do you get it? How does it work? What are the adverse effects? How well does it work? How long after unprotected sex can you take it? Does it work better when taken as soon as possible after unprotected sex, or does timing not matter? If there is no misinformation, the practitioner can congratulate the patient on her excellent level of knowledge and ask if she is willing to make sure that at least two friends learn about EC from her. The practitioner then can offer a prescription for Plan B or office-dispensed medication, if available, if the patient would like it.

If the patient is unable to answer any of the questions, the practitioner can ask the patient for permission to give her this information. If the patient has misinformation, the practitioner can ask the patient for permission to give her medically correct information that is different from what she has heard, because it might help her make better decisions for herself. If the patient agrees to receive the information, the practitioner can give her the medically accurate information about EC and then ask her, "What do you make of this new information?" and "How does this change anything for you?" If the patient does not give permission to receive information about EC, the practitioner can tell the patient, "You don't seem ready to hear more about this right now, but when you change your mind, I am always willing to give you medically accurate information about EC to help you make educated health decisions." The practitioner could also state, "I am not here to make you listen to a lecture or any information you are not interested in."

One common example of misinformation that occurs when the practitioner asks the patient to describe the way EC works is that many adolescents say, "It causes an abortion, miscarriage, or kills the baby." In this case, the practitioner can ask the patient to explain how a woman gets pregnant. If there is misinformation, the practitioner can ask permission to review with her the process by which a woman gets pregnant in terms of ovulation, fertilization, tubal transport, and implantation (using of a diagram with these stages is helpful). The practitioner can explain that EC works primarily by preventing ovulation (pointing to the ovary), but there is a possibility it might work some of the time by preventing the fertilized egg from sticking to the lining of the uterus (pointing to the picture of the egg implanting). The practitioner then can reinforce that once the egg sticks to the uterine lining and starts growing there (which we call a pregnancy), that EC will no longer work and will not unstick the pregnancy from the lining. The practitioner then can explain that unsticking the pregnancy from the uterine lining is called an abortion or a miscarriage. The practitioner then can ask if the way EC works is consistent with the patient's beliefs about ways that are acceptable to prevent pregnancy and ways that are not.

Summary

The available options for EC in the United States include POPs, with Plan B being the only dedicated product; COCs; and postcoital insertion of a copper-releasing IUD. Mifepristone is not available for use as EC in the United States.

For adolescents, the best EC choice is Plan B, given in a single dose within 120 hours of unprotected intercourse, but it may not be available at all pharmacies. Ovrette would be a good second choice, but cost may become a barrier, because two packages of pills are required. COCs may be used, but the two doses must be given 12 hours apart, and it is best to offer an antinausea medication to take 1 hour before the first dose. Rarely, an adolescent may have contraindications to using an estrogen-containing product, and in this case, Plan B also is preferred. The copper-releasing IUD can be considered for young women who are at low risk for STIs and who desire ongoing contraception from an IUD.

Until EC is available OTC for women of all ages, providers should attempt to make EC accessible to all adolescents who want it by educating patients and their partners about the method and giving an advance supply or prescription. Providers can supply adolescents with a list of pharmacies that are willing to dispense EC and enter into collaborative practice agreements, where legal, to improve access to this therapy.

References

[1] Martin JA, Hamilton BE, Sutton PD, et al. Births: final data for 2002. Natl Vital Stat Rep 2003;52(10):1–113.

[2] Singh S, Darroch JE. Adolescent pregnancy and childbearing: levels and trends in developed countries. Fam Plann Perspect 2000;32(1):14–23.

[3] Piccinino LJ, Mosher WD. Trends in contraceptive use in the United States: 1982–1995. Fam Plann Perspect 1998;30(1):4–10.

[4] Peterson LS, Oakley D, Potter LS, et al. Women's efforts to prevent pregnancy: consistency of oral contraceptive use. Fam Plann Perspect 1998;30(1):19–23.

[5] Henshaw SK. Unintended pregnancy in the United States. Fam Plann Perspect 1998;30(1):24–9.

[6] Stewart F, Trussell J, Van Look PF. Emergency contraception. In: Hatcher RA, Trussell J, Stewart F, et al, editors. Contraceptive technology. New York: Ardent Media; 2004. p. 279–303.

[7] von Hertzen H, Piaggio G, Ding J, et al. Low-dose mifepristone and two regimens of levonorgestrel for emergency contraception: a WHO multi-centre randomized trial. Lancet 2002; 360:1803–10.

[8] Ellertson C, Evans M, Ferden S, et al. Extending the time limit for starting the Yuzpe regimen of emergency contraception to 120 hours. Obstet Gynecol 2003;101(6):1168–71.

[9] Hatcher RA, Zieman M, Cwiak C, et al. A pocket guide to managing contraception. Tiger (GA): Bridging the Gap Foundation; 2004.

[10] Prescription drug products; certain combined oral contraceptives for use as postcoital emergency contraception. Fed Reg 1997;62(37):8609–12.

[11] Ellertson C, Webb A, Blanchard K, et al. Modifying the Yuzpe regimen of emergency contraception: a multi-center randomized controlled trial. Obstet Gynecol 2003;101(6):1160–7.

[12] Task Force on Postovulatory Methods of Fertility Regulation. Randomised controlled trial of levonorgestrel versus the Yuzpe regimen of combined oral contraceptives for emergency contraception. Lancet 1998;352:428–33.

[13] Piaggio G, von Hertzen H, Grimes DA, et al. Timing of emergency contraception with levonorgestrel or the Yuzpe regimen. Task Force on Postovulatory Methods of Fertility Regulation. Lancet 1999;353:721.

[14] Rodrigues I, Grou F, Joly J. Effectiveness of emergency contraceptive pills between 72 and 120 hours after unprotected sexual intercourse. Am J Obstet Gynecol 2001;184:531–7.

[15] Xiao B, Zhao H, Piaggio G, et al. Expanded clinical trial of emergency contraception with 10 mg mifepristone. Contraception 2003;68:431–7.

[16] Piaggio G, von Hertzen H, Heng Z, et al. Meta-analysis of randomized trials comparing different doses of mifepristone in emergency contraception. Contraception 2003;68:447–52.

[17] Trussell J, Ellertson C, von Hertzen H, et al. Estimating the effectiveness of emergency contraceptive pills. Contraception 2003;67:259–65.

[18] Raymond E, Taylor D, Trussell J, et al. Minimum effectiveness of the levonorgestrel regimen of emergency contraception. Contraception 2004;69:79–81.

[19] Romo LF, Berenson AB, Wu ZH. The role of misconceptions on Latino women's acceptance of emergency contraceptive pills. Contraception 2004;69:227–35.

[20] Croxatto HB, Oritz ME, Müller AL. Mechanisms of action of emergency contraception. Steroids 2003;68(10–13):1095–8.

[21] Marions L, Cekan SZ, Bygdeman M, et al. Effect of emergency contraception with levonorgestrel or mifepristone on ovarian function. Contraception 2004;69:373–7.

[22] Ortiz ME, Ortiz RE, Fuentes MA, et al. Postcoital administration of levonorgestrel does not interfere with postfertilization events in the new-world monkey Cebus apella. Hum Reprod 2004;19(6):1352–6.

[23] Trussell J, Ellertson C, Dorflinger L. Effectiveness of the Yuzpe regimen of emergency contraception by cycle day of intercourse: implications for mechanism of action. Contraception 2003;67:161–71.

[24] Thomas MA. Postcoital contraception. Clin Obstet Gynecol 2001;44(1):101–5.

[25] Mishell DR. Intrauterine devices: mechanisms of action, safety, and efficacy. Contraception 1998;58(3):45S–53S.

[26] Harper CC, Rocca CH, Darney PD, et al. Tolerability of levonorgestrel emergency contraception in adolescents. Am J Obstet Gynecol 2004;191:1158–63.

[27] Webb A, Shochet T, Bigrigg A, et al. Effect of hormonal emergency contraception on bleeding patterns. Contraception 2004;69:133–5.

[28] Piaggio G, Heng Z, von Hertzen H, et al. Combined effectiveness of mifepristone 10 mg in emergency contraception. Contraception 2003;68:439–46.

[29] Glasier A. Drug therapy: emergency postcoital contraception. N Engl J Med 1997;337(15):1058–64.

[30] Nielsen CL, Miller L. Ectopic gestation following emergency contraceptive pill administration. Contraception 2000;62:275–6.

[31] Gainer E, Méry C, Ulmann A. Letter to the editor. Contraception 2004;69:83–4.

[32] Bissell P, Anderson C. Supplying emergency contraception via community pharmacies in the UK: reflections on the experiences of users and providers. Soc Sci Med 2003;57(12):2367–78.

[33] Glasier A, Baird D. The effects of self-administering emergency contraception. N Engl J Med 1998;339(1):1–4.

[34] Lovvorn A, Nerquaye-Tetteh J, Glover EK, et al. Provision of emergency contraceptive pills to spermicide users in Ghana. Contraception 2000;61:287–93.

[35] Ellertson C, Ambardekar S, Hedley A, et al. Emergency contraception: randomized comparison of advance provision and information only. Obstet Gynecol 2001;98(4):570–5.

[36] Jackson RA, Schwarz EB, Freedman L, et al. Advance supply of emergency contraception: effect on use and usual contraception—a randomized trial. Obstet Gynecol 2003;102(1):8–16.

[37] Lo SST, Fan SYS, Ho PC, et al. Effect of advanced provision of emergency contraception on women's contraceptive behaviour: a randomized controlled trial. Hum Reprod 2004;19(10): 2404–10.

[38] Raine T, Harper C, Leon K, et al. Emergency contraception: advance provision in a young, high-risk clinic population. Obstet Gynecol 2000;96:1–7.

[39] Gold MA, Wolford JE, Smith KA, et al. The effects of advance provision of emergency contraception on adolescent women's sexual and contraceptive behaviors. J Pediatr Adolesc Gynecol 2004;17:87–96.

[40] Raine TR, Harper CC, Rocca CH, et al. Direct access to emergency contraception through pharmacies and effect on contraception and STIs: a randomized controlled trial. JAMA 2005; 293:54–62.

[41] Conard LE, Gold MA. Emergency contraceptive pills: a review of the recent literature. Curr Opin Obstet Gynecol 2004;16:389–95.

[42] Gold MA, Sucato G, Conard LE, et al. Provision of emergency contraception to adolescents: position paper of the Society for Adolescent Medicine. J Adolesc Health 2004;35:66–70.

[43] Conard LA, Fortenberry JD, Blythe MJ, et al. Pharmacists' attitudes and toward and practices with adolescents. Arch Pediatr Adolesc Med 2003;157(4):361–5.

[44] Bennett W, Petraitis C, D'Anella A, et al. Pharmacists' knowledge and the difficulty of obtaining emergency contraception. Contraception 2003;68(4):261–7.

[45] Espey E, Ogburn T, Howard D, et al. Emergency contraception: pharmacy access in Albuquerque, New Mexico. Obstet Gynecol 2003;102(5, Part 1):918–21.

[46] The Alan Guttmacher Institute. State policies in brief. New York: Alan Guttmacher Institute; 2004.

[47] Rollnick S, Miller WR. What is motivational interviewing? Behavioral and Cognitive Psychotherapy 1995;23:325–34.

[48] Miller WR, Rollnick, editors. Motivational interviewing. Preparing people for change. 2nd edition. New York: Guilford Press; 2002.

[49] Rollnick S, Mason P, Butler C, editors. Health behavior change: a guide for practitioners. London: Churchill Livingstone; 1999.

Further readings

1–888-NOT-2-LATE.

http://www.backupyourbirthcontrol.org. Web site about emergency contraception.

www.managingcontraception.com.Web site with information about emergency contraception.

www.NOT-2-LATE.com. Web site about emergency contraception and how to find providers who will prescribe it.

ELSEVIER
SAUNDERS

ADOLESCENT
MEDICINE
CLINICS

Adolesc Med 16 (2005) 603–616

Natural Contraception

Cora Collette Breuner, MD, MPH

Adolescent Medicine Section, Department of Pediatrics, Children's Hospital and Medical Center,
4800 Sand Point Way NE, Seattle, WA 98105, USA

Among consumers and health professionals, complementary and alternative medicine (CAM) has become sought after and integrated into mainstream provision of medical services. CAM, known as nonallopathic, unconventional, holistic, or natural therapy, encompasses many types of healing practices [1,2] From the Cochrane Collaboration, CAM is a "a broad domain of healing resources that encompasses all health systems, modalities, and practices and their accompanying theories and beliefs, other than those intrinsic to the politically dominant health systems in a particular society or culture in a given historical period" [3].

A 1993 Harvard study documented that in 1990, more than one-third of Americans used unconventional therapies [4]. In a second study, this number increased by 38%, from 60 million to 83 million people per year between 1990 and 1997. Expenditures for visits to alternative medicine providers were estimated at $21.2 billion, $12.2 billion of which was paid out-of-pocket. Nearly one in five individuals taking prescription medicines also was taking herbs or high-dose vitamin supplements [5]. CAM use is considerably higher in specific groups of children and adolescents, such as in those with cystic fibrosis, cancer, arthritis, and in those undergoing surgery [6–12]. Use in homeless adolescents was noted to be 70% and was felt to be caused, among other things, by a need to use something natural and a mistrust of mainstream health care. These youth faced medical and mental health illness on an acute and chronic basis yet felt more confidence in a system that embraces CAM [13]. From a Detroit study, 12% of the pediatric patients were using CAM [14]. A significant predictor for CAM use in the pediatric populations is the use of CAM by parents.

Primary care providers are resources for advice and recommendations about using CAM. Adult primary care providers maintain an open attitude toward CAM

E-mail address: cora.breuner@seattlechildrens.org

and may make referrals to CAM providers, or use CAM themselves [15–21]. Similar findings were seen within a study of pediatricians [22].

There are multiple effective contraceptive medical allopathic choices available for women and men in the form of the birth control pill, injectables, barrier methods, intrauterine devices, and sterilization. Yet these may not be the only options that people use, as made clear from studies on CAM use. The contracepting community, of which adolescents may be active or passive members, includes those who seek alternative choices for many chronic illnesses, for prevention or health maintenance, and as an adjunct to the medical services provided by allopathic providers. This article discusses some of these options for contraception, including natural family planning and plant- derived hormonal contraception. The discussion will include medical evidence to support or refute these methods, potential dangers of these interventions, and additional resources for those who want to learn more.

Natural family planning—historical view

The concept of regulating fertility is not a new one. The decline in fertility among the white middle class was noted in Europe and then the United States in the 19th century [23]. The gospel of self sovereignty and fewer children and healthy, happy maternity was coincident with reproductive control and drew considerable support around the time of the Civil War. Fertile times, when sexual activity needed to be curtailed, were documented in diaries and in the medical literature and were discussed at length in the higher social circles.

Family planning has belonged to a highly discordant and not necessarily peaceable clan [24,25]. Family planning to many has been the cornerstone of feminism, redefining the role of women from their patriarchal-defined role as child bearers and household managers. For others, the term is synonymous with abortion. The criminalization of abortion during the latter half of the 19th century drove reproductive services and dissemination of information underground until the middle of the 20th century. Only recently has it become apparent that discussion of contraception is less of a taboo and more of an ethical right for women and men.

From the historical perspective in island and native cultures, sexual taboos against premarital and adolescent sexual union did not exist, as observed and recorded by anthropologists. One reviewer noted that in these cultures where sexual experimentation among adolescents was allowed, there was a general absence of pregnancy [26]. Ethnographic reports are highlighted in the next section.

Regarding the Triobriand islanders in Oceania

> Since there is so much sexual freedom, must there not be a great number of children born out of wedlock? If this is not so, what means of prevention do the natives employ? . . .it is very remarkable to note that illegitimate children are

rare. The girls seem to remain sterile throughout their period of license...until they marry; when they are married they conceive and breed sometimes quite prolifically...I was able to find roughly a dozen illegitimate children recorded genealogically throughout Triobriands, or about 1%. Thus we are faced with the questions: why are there so few illegitimate children? ...they never practice coitus interruptus [27].

In the textbook *Medical History of Contraception,* Himes postulated that desire for contraception is a universal social phenomenon; every society possesses some knowledge of birth control, even if the methods are not always effective. Ethnographers in the era along with Himes rejected the idea of medicinal plants, roots, and barks as commonly used contraceptives. Female researchers who visited these cultures, however, were able to establish trust with the native women in Peru, the Pacific islands, and the Pacific Northwest Native American Shoshone and learned of contraceptive plants grown in small secret gardens and used by these indigenous women.

The questions from the past remain pertinent today. Women want to know: when am I the most fertile? When am I the least fertile? And for adolescents, what is the perfect (easiest) way to keep from getting pregnant? (tonight)? For many, natural birth control answers these questions and helps women to be more in control of their fertility.

In the United States, approximately 4% of women of reproductive age use natural family planning (NFP) to avoid pregnancy. In one study, a questionnaire was mailed to 1500 women, aged 18 to 50 in Missouri in 1992. Almost 25% stated that they would probably use NFP in the future to avoid pregnancy, and 37.4% indicated that they would likely use NFP in the future to become pregnant [28]. A woman's decision regarding her desires for a family are planted well before her actual first pregnancy, most likely during her adolescent years [29]. Women are seeking out information on natural birth control as a method to prevent pregnancy [30].

Can adolescents learn information needed for natural family planning?

The correspondence of cervical mucorrhea with elevated concentrations of serum and 24-hour urinary estrogens has been established [31–33]. Can this information be disseminated to the adolescent population? Many would think that this is a concept far from the grasp of an adolescent. Yet Klaus and Martin evaluated this and concluded that ethnically and socioeconomically diverse perimenarchal girls can be taught to recognize their cervical mucus patterns and distinguish anovulatory from ovulatory cycles [34].

Young women can take an interest in the physiology of their own bodies. In a study on the pathophysiology of polycystic ovarian syndrome, women performed menstrual charting in an attempt to understand ovulatory disorders. Although this article focused on polycystic ovary syndrome and hypothalamic dysfunction, information gained from a paper such as this can be used in future research on the reproductive health education of the young woman. With knowledge of fertility

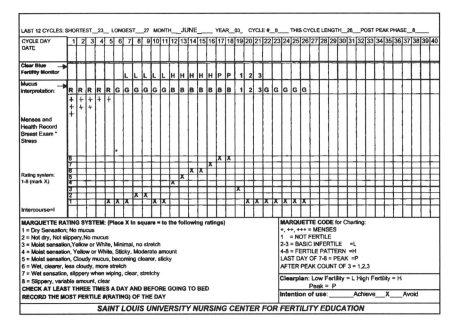

Fig. 1. Marquette model chart. Most commonly patients color code the interpretation: red for menses, green for infertile day, blue for fertile day. The amount of flow is also described is the space allotted for comments. This chart represents a luteal phase deficiency. Note the shortened luteal phase of only 8 days. (*From:* Barron ML. Proactive management of menstrual cycle abnormalities in young women. J Perinat Neonat Nurs 2004;18(2):81–92.)

and menstrual cycle function, adolescents and young women are in a stronger position to make informed decisions about how they wish to manage their reproductive and sexual health [35].

There are many types of NFP, including the Billings Method (the ovulation or mucous method), named for Australian doctors Jon and Evelyn Billings. This method charts the presence and description of cervical fluid [36]. The mucous method describes three different cervical fluids during the menstrual cycle: (1) sticky, tacky, and dry occurring after menstruation, (2) creamy, milky, and smooth, which occurs right before the most fertile period, which is (3) slippery, egg white, stretchable, clear, and yellow /pink or red tinged. Women are taught to avoid intravaginal sexual activity when the cervical mucous reflects the most fertile time [37]. An example of this method is noted in Fig. 1.

Herbal contraception

Herbal products historically have been the cornerstone of much of the pharmaceutical armamentarium. Active segments of the plant include leaves, flowers, stems, roots, seeds, and berries. Plant-derived products used by health care pro-viders include the statins, which are derived from the fungus *Aspergillus terreus*; cephalosporins, derived from a marine fungus (*Cephalosporium acremonium*); digoxin from foxglove (*Digitalis lanata*), progesterone (*Dioscorea villosa,* Mexican yam); and cromolyn sodium, a khellin derivative from the Ayurvedic herb *Ammi visnaga* [38].

From the Harvard studies on CAM use in 1990 and 1997, the use of self-prescribed herbal remedies within the United States increased from 2.5% to 12.1% [4,5]. The proportion of individuals consulting practitioners of herbal medicine rose from 10.2% to 15.1%, and they spent around $5 billion on herbal medicines. In 1998, Brevoort estimated the total retail sales of herbal medicines close to $4 billion [39].

Experts in the field of naturopathy and medicine do not support herbal contraception because of the lack of scientific evidence of efficacy and the pos-sibility of adverse outcomes. With that in mind, it is known that the plant king-dom contains numerous bioactive substances that may affect the regulation of reproduction. Many herbs have been used to reduce fertility with little or no scientific evidence supporting this claim [40]. Berman, an expert in CAM, does not recommend contraceptive herbs in that they may be abortifacients that work by poisoning the woman [41]. Fifty-seven poisonings from attempts at herbal abortion, including two deaths, were reported in a 1900 to 1997 review [42]. The German Commission E Monographs issued repeated warnings that many herbs can cause pregnancy termination as a side effect and so are not recommended in the pregnant patient or in one desiring pregnancy [43]. Importantly, many of these herbal supplements may be substandard both in content of active constituents and in lack of contamination. Health professionals need to educate their patients on the lack of stringent federal regulation of these products. There have been recent attempts at improving the standards [44,45].

The following herbs and other compounds have been evaluated predominantly in the laboratory with mixed results. If available, information on typical doses is cited. Techniques used for extraction of the bioactive ingredients of these herbs are noted to use ethanol or methanol, which may cause some of the anticontraceptive effects. Except for the isolated occasion, many of these herbs have not been studied in people. Despite this, usage may be higher in women and men than previously thought judging by the high volume of people accessing herbal contraception on the Internet (eg, www.sisterzeus.com). It is not known how many adolescents use these products.

Ovulation inhibition, anti-implantation

Queen Anne's lace seeds/Wild carrot (Daucus carota)

Women have used seeds from *Daucus carota* for centuries; the earliest written references dates back to the late 5th century BC appearing in a work written by Hippocrates. Many view Queen Anne's lace as a promising postcoital agent, and Internet discussion recommends use similar to emergency contraception, although there has been little or no scientific evidence to support this claim. Typically, one teaspoon of the seeds are chewed and then swallowed with water or juice. The claim is that the volatile oils from the seeds prevent implantation, and thus the seeds must be chewed before swallowing [46].

Stem bark extracts

Multiple studies on the stem bark extracts of *Combretodendron macrocarpum, Cola nitida, Afrormosia laxiflora,* and *Pterocarpus erinaceus* have shown that they block the estrus cycle of female rats. It is thought that these compounds may bind to steroid receptor sites with resultant antigonadotropic activity. The most potent competitor for steroid receptors was *C macrocarpum* extract, followed by *P erinaceus, C nitida* and *A laxiflora* [47–49].

Rivea plant *(*Rivea hypocrateriformis*)*

The plant *Rivea hypocrateriformis* was tested for anti-implantation effects and as an abortifacient in female rats using petroleum ether, chloroform, ethanol, and distilled water extracts. The ethanol extract was found to be most effective in causing significant anti-implantation and interruption of early pregnancy. The active ethanol extract contained alkaloids, glycosides, saponins, tannins, and phenolic compounds. Whether the contraceptive effects of this plant are caused by the constituents of the extract or an active ingredient of the plant is unclear [50].

Castor plant *(*Ricinus communis*)*

This plant is a native of India with 17 species that produce large seeds containing the active constituent ricin, a glycoprotein. The castor oil from the seed has been used as a purgative and traditionally is accepted as a contraceptive by women throughout India and Africa. Ricin also is found in smartweed leaves *(Polygonum hydropiper)*. In a study looking at mechanism of action of this compound, female laboratory animals were injected with ricin, placed in cages with males of the same species and then had laparotomies looking for fetus implantation. Controls were injected with estradiol. The findings from this study indicated that *Ricinus communis* might possess estrogenic and anti-implantation activity [51].

Contraception was evaluated in people using the seeds of *Ricinus communis* (RICOM-1013-J) in two separate studies. In both trials, women were given one single oral dose of 2.3 to 2.5 g. No pregnancies were detected in subjects for 1 year in one study and for 8 months in the second study. Adverse effects included headache, nausea, vomiting, weight gain, loss of appetite, increased blood pressure, and dysmenorrhea. The results of the liver and renal function profiles in women volunteers showed that there were no significant $(P < .05)$ changes in renal functions on day 206 following RICOM-1013-J administration. Serum levels of alkaline phosphatase and GGT, however, showed a slight rise in about 70% of volunteers, whereas bilirubin and transaminases levels were normal [52,53]. There was no documentation of use of other forms of contraception during the study period. Ricin contained in the outer hull of the castor seed is considered possibly effective as a contraceptive when taken as a single oral dose as noted in Natural Medicine Comprehensive Database [54,55]. The oil from the seeds has been used by midwives to induce labor; for this reason, it should not be used in women who are pregnant and are not at term, as it may induce miscarriage.

*Wild yam (*Dioscorea villosa*)*

It has been hypothesized that wild yam contains dehydroepiandrosterone-like properties and may act as a precursor to estrogen and progesterone. In the 1960s, progesterone, androgens, and cortisone were chemically manufactured from Mexican wild yam, and this has led many to believe consumption of this plant can lead to the same chemical conversion in the human body. It is used for dysmenorrhea and as an alternative to hormone replacement therapy to treat the symptoms of menopause [56]. It is not recommended as a contraceptive agent [57].

*Marshmallow plant (*Malvaviscus conzattii*)*

The methanol extract of the flowers of *Malvaviscus conzattii* was administered to rats orally and was found to be effective in inhibiting ovulation. From these data, the researchers suggested that there might be an interference with the synthesis or release of gonadotropins from the pituitary gland [58].

*Asparagus (*Asparagus pubescens*)*

The methanolic extract of *Asparagus pubescens* root was investigated for its contraceptive activity in mice, rats, and rabbits. Fetal implantation was inhibited in a dose-dependent manner [59].

Other herbs

In India, many antifertility herbs are used by indigenous peoples living in the hills (*Drynaria quercifolia*) [60]. Ayurvedic traditional herbs are used by those in more urban environments (*Pippaliyadi vati, Molluga stricta, Ruta graveolens, Derris brevipes* variety *coriace*). Studies are preliminary on mechanism of action and efficacy of these herbs [61–64]. In one laboratory study using *Ferula jaeschkeana*, uterine implantation was inhibited by ingesting an extract of this herb [65]. Similar studies of Ethiopian indigenous medicinal plants traditionally used as antifertility agents appear in the literature [66].

Abortifacient

Every indigenous pharmacopeia contains some type of herbal abortifacient, and these plant products are among the oldest of herbal medicines. Anecdotal evidence suggests that use of herbal abortifacients declines when safe, legal, and affordable clinical abortion and contraception is available.

*Pennyroyal (*Hedoema pulegiodes*)*

Pennyroyal traditionally has been used as an abortifacient, yet its toxicity is well documented [67,68]. Doses required for abortion can cause irreversible kidney damage, hepatic disease, and death. It is not recommended and is considered unsafe by Natural Medicine Comprehensive Database.

In a retrospective study of 86 cases of herbal infusion ingestion with abortive intent reported to the Poison Control Center Uruguay between 1986 and 1999, 35 plant names representing 30 species were used. Most frequently used were rue (ruda; *Ruta graveolens*), cola de quirquincho (*Lycopodium saururus*), a type of parsley (*Petroselinum hortense*), and an over-the-counter herbal product called Carachipita, which contains pennyroyal (*Mentha pulegium*), yerba de la perdiz (*Margiricarpus pinnatus*), oregano (*Origanum vulgare*), and guaycurú (*Statice brasiliensis*). In 23 cases, patients ingested homemade brews made from two to six different species. Rue and parsley were among the more successful abortion agents; they were also among those producing the most toxic symptoms [69].

Spermicidal

Sedum praealtum

Intravaginal ethanol extracts of *Sedum praealtum* in mice decrease spermatozoa viability for 24 hours after administration [70].

Cotton plant (Gossypium hirsutum)

Gossypol has been studied in women as an effective spermicide and has been found to immobilize spermatozoa when inserted intravaginally. It also has been shown to have an inhibitory effect on herpes simplex virus in vitro [71].

Neem oil (Azardirachta indica)

Neem oil pressed from the bark of *Azardirachta indica*, a native Indian plant, is considered a spermicidal agent when used intravaginally. It also has antimicrobial and antifungal properties [72]. Orally, neem oil caused arrest of spermatogenesis in male rats along with a decrease in sperm motility and density [73]. Intrauterine neem oil administered to rats and monkeys caused a block in fetal implantation [74].

Zinc acetate and Aloe barbadensis

In a study using 20 samples of fresh ejaculate from volunteers (age 20 to 30 years), zinc acetate was noted to be spermicidal. Lyophilized *Aloe barbadensis* also was noted to be spermicidal because of the spermatozoa tail toxicity from multiple elements present in small amounts (boron, barium, calcium, chromium, copper, iron, potassium, magnesium, manganese, phosphorus, and zinc). In the laboratory animal, these compounds did not irritate the vaginal epithelium. It was suggested that zinc acetate and lyophilized *Aloe barbadensis* warranted further study as a vaginal contraceptive [75].

Male antifertility herbs

Cotton plant (Gossypium *hirsutum*)

Gossypol (*Gossypium hirsutum*) is a polyphenolic extract of the seed of the cotton plant, and, when taken orally, it may suppress sperm concentration by inhibiting spermatogenesis [76,77]. Gossypol can cause fatigue, hypokalemia, persistent oligospermia. and can interfere with digoxin or other diuretics. It typically is taken as 15–20 mg/d [78].

*Papaya (*Carica papaya*)*

Papaya has been used as a male contraceptive. In adult male rabbits receiving an aqueous extract of papaya seeds orally, no contraceptive effects were noted contrary to the observations made in previous studies [79].

Piperine

Piperine has been used as an oral male contraceptive agent. Histological studies in male rats receiving piperine revealed a partial degeneration of germ cell types, damage to the seminiferous tubule, decrease in seminiferous tubular and Leydig cell nuclear diameter, and desquamation of spermatocytes and spermatids. A 10 mg dose of piperine caused a marked increase in serum gonadotropins and a decrease in intratesticular testosterone concentration. The clinical implications of this study are unclear [80].

Nicotine

Nicotine causes a reduction in the weight of epididymis and vas deferens in rat studies. The clinical implications of this finding are unclear [81].

*Thunder god vine (*Lei Gong Teng*)*

Thunder god vine has been used for rheumatoid arthritis, menorrhagia, multiple sclerosis, and as a male contraceptive. There is insufficient evidence of efficacy for use as a male contraceptive, but it is postulated that in thunder god leaf and root, the triptolide and tripdiolide inhibit sperm transformation, maturation, and motility. Fertility may return to normal 6 weeks after cessation of use. Adverse effects include gastrointestinal upset, diarrhea, headache, hair loss, and immunosuppression [82].

Tripterygium hypoglaucum

Tripterygium hypoglaucum is a plant used in southern China for renal, liver, skin, and rheumatoid diseases. It also is considered a male antifertility herb. In 24 males aged 20 to 43 years who were given a daily concoction for 2 to 48 months, sperm motility and concentration were lower than in control subjects. These sperm changes were reversed 6 to 12 months after cessation of treatment. Follicle-stimulating hormone, luteinizing hormone, testosterone levels, and libido were similar in treated and control groups [83].

Solanum xanthocarpum

Solanum xanthocarpum is being studied in the laboratory in India as an inhibitor of spermatogenesis [84].

Anacardium occidentale

β-sitosterol, a phytosterol isolated from the leaves of *Anacardium occidentale*, can cause estrogenic effects and reduce the number of implantation sites in rabbits [85]. It also can inhibit the process of spermatogenesis in male rats [86]. Two doses were studied in rats for 16, 32, and 48 days. High-dose treatment reduced sperm concentration and weights of testis. Further studies were recommended [87].

Summary

The field of CAM is broad and diverse [88–90]. CAM therapies may be viewed as an adjunct to conventional treatment or as a primary source of medical service [91,92]. Understanding patient choices, and supporting them if safe, reflect respect for the health care choices made by patients [93]. Health care providers must be aware of the safety and efficacy of alternative treatments and know how to access resources to help guide the patient methodically through a decision tree on CAM use for contraception.

References

[1] Spigelblatt LS. Alternative medicine: should it be used by children? Curr Probl Pediatr 1995;25: 180–8.

[2] Breuner CC. Complementary medicine in pediatrics: a review of acupuncture, homeopathy, massage and chiropractic therapies. Current Probl Pediatr Adolesc Health Care 2002;32(10): 347–84.

[3] Zollman C, Vickers A. What is complementary medicine? BMJ 1999;319:393–6.

[4] Eisenberg DM, Kessler RC, Foster C, et al. Unconventional medicine in the United States. N Engl J Med 1993;328:246–52.

[5] Eisenberg DM, Davis RB, Ettner SL, et al. Trends in alternative medicine use in the United States, 1990–1997. JAMA 1998;280:1569–75.

[6] Stem RC, Canda ER, Doershuk CF. Use of nonmedical treatment by cystic fibrosis patients. J Adolesc Health 1992;13:612–5.

[7] Sawyer MG, Gannoni AF, Toogood IR, et al. The use of alternatives therapies by children with cancer. Med J Aust 1994;169:320–2.

[8] Southwood TR, Malleson PN, Roberts-Thomson PJ, et al. Unconventional remedies used by patients with juvenile arthritis. Pediatrics 1995;85:150–4.

[9] Neuhouser ML, Patterson RE, Schwartz SM, et al. Use of alternative medicine by children with cancer in Washington State. Prev Med 2001;33(5):347–54.

[10] Friedman T, Slayton WB, Allen LS, et al. Use of alternative therapies for children with cancer. Pediatrics 1997;100(6):E1.

[11] Faw C, Ballentine R, Ballentine L, et al. Unproved cancer remedies. A survey of use in pediatric outpatients. JAMA 1977;238:1536–8.

[12] Paramore LC. Use of alternative therapies: estimates from the Robert Wood Johnson Foundation national access to care survey, US Cancer Pain Relief Committee. J Pain Symptom Manage 1997;13:83–9.

[13] Breuner CC, Barry P, Kemper KJ. Alternative medicine use by homeless youth. Arch Pediatr Adolesc Med 1998;152(11):1071–5.

[14] Sawni-Sikand A, Schubiner H, Thomas RL. Use of complementary/alternative therapies among children in primary care pediatrics. Ambul Pediatr 2002;2(2):99–103.

[15] Burg MA, Kosch S, Neims A. Personal use of alternative medicine therapies by health science faculty. JAMA 1998;280:1563.

[16] Borkan J, Neher JO, Anson O, Smoker B. Referrals for alternative therapies. J Fam Pract 1994; 39:545–50.

[17] Blumberg DL, Grant WD, Hendricks SR, et al. The physician and unconventional medicine. Altern Ther Health Med 1995;1:31–5.

[18] Berman BM, Singh BK, Lao L, et al. Physicians' attitudes toward complementary or alternative medicine: a regional survey. J Am Board Fam Pract 1995;8:361–6.

[19] Verhoef MJ, Sutherland LR. Alternative medicine and general practitioners: opinions and behavior. Can Fam Physician 1995;41:1005–11.

[20] Boucher TA, Lenz SK. An organizational survey of physicians: attitudes about and practice of complementary and alternative medicine. Alternative Therapies 1998;4:59–64.

[21] Committee on Children with Disabilities. Counseling families who chose CAM for their child with chronic illness or disability. Pediatrics 2001;107(3):598–601.

[22] Sikand A, Laken M. Pediatricians' experience with and attitudes toward complementary/ alternative medicine. Arch Pediatr Adolesc Med 1998;152:1059–64.

[23] Brodie JF. Contraception and abortion in 19th century America. Ithaca (NY): Cornell University; 1994.

[24] Maguire DC. Sacred choices: the right to contraception and abortion in ten world religions. Minneapolis (MN): Fortress Press; 2001.

[25] Hilgers TW. The medical applications of natural family planning. Omaha (NE): Pope Paul VI Institute Press; 1991.

[26] De Meo J. The use of contraceptive plant materials by native peoples. The Journal of Orgonomy 1992;26(1):152–76.

[27] Malinowski B. The sexual life of savages in N.W. Melanesia. London: Routledge and Keegan Paul; 1929.

[28] Stanford JB, Lemaire JC, Thurman PB. Women's interest in natural family planning. J Fam Pract 1998;46(1):65–71.

[29] Kass-Annese B, Danzer H. Natural birth control. Alameda (CA): Hunter House; 2003.

[30] Dworkin N. What you may not know about natural birth control. Vegetarian times. Alt Health Watch 1998;251:82–91.

[31] Barron ML, Daly KD. Expert in fertility appreciation: the Creighton model practitioner. J Obstet Gynecol Neonatal Nurs 2001;30:386–91.

[32] Fehring RJ. Accuracy of the peak day of cervical mucus as a biological marker of fertility. Contraception 2002;66:231–5.

[33] Guida M, Tommaselli GA, Palomba S, et al. Efficacy of methods for determining ovulation in a natural family planning program. Fertil Steril 1999;72:900–4.

[34] Klaus H, Martin JL. Recognition of ovulatory/ anovulatory cycle patterns in adolescents by mucus self-detection. J Adolesc Health Care 1989;10:93–6.

[35] Barron ML. Proactive management of menstrual cycle abnormalities in young women. J Perinat Neonat Nurs 2004;18(2):81–92.

[36] Billings Ovulation Method Association. Available at: www.boma~usa.org. Accessed July 12, 2005.

[37] Weschler T. Taking charge of your fertility: the definitive guide to natural birth control, pregnancy achievement and reproductive health. New York: Harper Collins; 2002.

[38] Rotblatt M, Ziment I. Evidence-based herbal medicine. Philadelphia: Hanley and Belfus; 2002.

[39] Brevoort P. The booming US botanical market: a new overview. HerbalGram 1998;44:33–48.

[40] Hudson T. Women's encyclopedia of natural medicine. Lincolwood (IL): Keats Publishing; 1999.

[41] Fugh- Berman A. Herbal birth control. Natural Health 2002;32(1):38.

[42] Ko RJ. Causes, epidemiology and clinical evaluation of suspected herbal poisoning. J Toxicol Clin Toxicol 1999;37(6):697–708.

[43] Blumenthal M, Busse WR, Goldberg A, et al. The complete German Commission E monographs: therapeutic Guide to Herbal Medicines. Boston: American Botanical Council; 1998.

[44] Dvorkin L, Gardiner PM. Regulation of dietary supplements in the United States of America. Clinical Research and Regulatory Affairs 2003;20(3):313–25.

[45] McGuffin M, Hobbs C, Upton R, et al, editors. Botanical safety handbook. New York: CRC Press; 1997.

[46] The contraceptive properties of carrots. Available at: website.lineone.net/~stolarczyk/cont.html. Accessed December 17, 2004.

[47] Benie T, El Izzi A, Tahiri C, et al. *Combretodendron africanum* bark extract as an antifertility agent. I: estrogenic effects in vivo and LH release by cultured gonadotrope cells. J Ethnopharmacol 1990;29(1):13–23.

[48] Benie T, Duval J, Thieulant ML. Effects of some traditional plant extracts on rat estrous cycle compared with Clomid. Phototherapy Research 2003;17(7):748–55.

[49] El Izzi A, Benie T, Thieulant ML, et al. Inhibitory effects of saponins from *Tetrapleura tetraptera* on the LH released by cultured rat pituitary cells. Planta Med 1990;56(4):357–9.

[50] Shivalingappa H, Satyanaran ND, Pirohit MG. Anti-implantation and pregnancy interruption efficacy of *Rivea hypocrateriformis* in the rat. J Ethnopharmacol 2001;74(3):245–9.

[51] Okwuasaba FK, Osunkwo UA, Ekwenchi MM, et al. Anticonceptive and estrogenic effects of seed extract of *Ricinus communis* var. minor. J Ethnopharmacol 1991;34:141–5.

[52] Ishchei CO, Das SC, Ogunkeye OO, et al. Preliminary clinical investigation of the contraceptive efficacy and chemical pathological effects of RICOM-1013 J of *Ricinus communis* car Minor on women volunteers. Phototherapy Research 2000;14(1):40–2.

[53] Das SC, Ischei CO, Okwuasaba FK, et al. Parry O Chemical, pathological and toxicological studies of the effects of RICOM-1013-J of Ricinus communis var Minor on women volunteers and rodents. Phytother Res 2000;14(1):15–9.

[54] Der Marderosian A. Review of Natural Products by Facts and Comparisons. St. Louis (MO): Kluker Publishing; 1999.

[55] Gruenwald J, Brendler T, Jaenicke C. PDR for herbal medicines. Montvale (NJ): Medical Economics Co.; 1998.

[56] Russell L, Hicks GS, Low AK, et al. Phytoestrogens: a viable option? Am J Med Sci 2002; 324(4):185–8.

[57] Basch E, Ulbricht C, Sollars D, et al. Wild yam (*Dioscoreaceae*). J Herb Pharmacother 2003; 3(4):77–91.

[58] Banaree R, Pal AK, Kabir SN, et al. Antiovulatory faculty of the flower of *Malvaviscus conzatti*. Phytother Res 1999;13(2):169–71.

[59] Nwafor PA, Owusaba FK, Onoruvwe OO. Contraceptive and nonestrogenic effects of methanolic extract of Asparagus pubescens root in experimental animals. J Ethnopharmacol 1998;62(2):117–22.

[60] Rajendran A, Rajan S. *Drynaria quercifolia*—an antifertility agent. Ancient Science of Life 1996;15(4):286–7.

[61] Chaudhury MR, Chandrasekaran R, Michra S. Embryotoxicity and teratogenicity studies of an ayruvedic contraceptive—*Pippaliyadi vati*. J Ethnopharmacol 2001;74(2):189–93.

[62] Padma P, Khosa RL. Identity of *Mollugo stricta* roots: a potential antifertility drug for future. Ancient Science of Life 1995;15(2):97–101.

[63] Gandhi M, Lal R, Sankaranarayanan A, et al. Postcoital antifertility activity of *Ruta graveolens* in female rats and hamsters. J Ethnopharmacol 1991;34(1):49–59.

[64] Badami S, Aneesh R, Sankar S, et al. Antifertility activity of *Derris brevipes* variety coriacea. J Ethnopharmacol 2003;84(1):99–104.

[65] Prakash AO, Pathak S, Mathur R. Postcoital contraceptive action in rats of a hexane extract of the aerial parts of *Ferula jaeschkeana*. J Ethnopharmacol 1991;34:221–34.

[66] Desta B. Ethiopian traditional herbal drugs. Part III: antifertility activity of 70 medicinal plants. J Ethnopharmacol 1994;44(3):199–209.

[67] Anderson IB, Meeker JE, Mullen WH, et al. Pennyroyal toxicity: measurement of toxic metabolite in two cases and review of the literature. Ann Intern Med 1996;124:726–34.

[68] Sullivan JB, Rumack BH, Thomas H, et al. Pennyroyal oil poisoning and hepatotoxicity. JAMA 1979;242:2873–4.

[69] Ciganda C, LcBorde A. Herbal infusions used for abortion. Journal Toxicology 2003;41(3):235–9.

[70] Silva-Torres R, Montellano-Rosales H, Ramos-Zamora D, et al. Spermicidal activity of the crude ethanol extract *Sedum praealtum* in mice. J Ethnopharmacol 2003;85(1):15–7.

[71] Ratsula K, Haukkamaa M, Wichmann K, et al. Vaginal contraception with Gossypol: a clinical study. Contraception 1983;27(6):571–6.

[72] SaiRam M, Ilvavazhagan G, Sharma SK, et al. Antimicrobial activity of a new vaginal contraceptive NIM-76 from neem oil (*Azardirachta indica*). J Ethnopharmacol 2000;71(3):377–82.

[73] Purohit O. Antifertility efficacy of neem bark (*Azadirachta indica* Aa. Juss) in male rats. Ancient Science of Life 1999;19(2):21–4.

[74] Garg S, Talwar GP, Upahdhayay SN. Immunocontraceptive activity guided fractionation and characterization for active constituent of neem (*Azadirachta induca*) seed extracts. J Ethnopharmacol 1998;60(3):235–46.

[75] Fahim MS, Wang M. Zinc acetate and lyophilized *Aloe barbadensis* as vaginal contraceptive. Contraception 1996;53:231–6.

[76] Natural Medicines Comprehensive Data. Available at: www.naturaldatabase.com/(wn315qbn mryxp45j3b4pvjd). Accessed December 8, 2004.

[77] Countinho EM, Athayde C, Alta G, et al. Gossypol blood levels and inhibition of spermatogenesis in men taking Gossypol as a contraceptive. A multi-center, international, dose- finding study. Contraception 2000;61(1):61–7.

[78] Wu D. An overview of the clinical pharmacology and therapeutic potential of Gossypol as a male contraceptive agent and in gynecological disease. Drugs 1989;38(3):333–41.

[79] Lohiya NK, Pathak N, Mishra PK, et al. Contraceptive evaluation and toxicological study of aqueous seed extract of the seeds of Carica papaya in male rabbits. J Ethnopharmacol 2000;70(1):17–27.

[80] Malini T, Manimaran RR, Arunakan J, et al. Effects of piperine on testis of albino rats. J Ethnopharmocol 1999;64(3):219–25.

[81] Londonkar RL, Srincaraseddy P, Somanathreddy P, et al. Nicotine-induced inhibition of the activities of accessory reproductive ducts in male rats. J Ethnopharmacol 1998;60(3):215–21.

[82] Natural Medicines Comprehensive Data. Available at: www.naturaldatabase.com. Accessed December 6, 2004.

[83] Qian SZ, et al. Effects of *Tripterygium hypoglaucum* (Levl. Hutch) on male fertility. Adv Contracept 1988;4:307–10.

[84] Purohit A. Contraceptive efficacy of *Solanum xanthocarpum* berry in male rats. Ancient Science of Life 1992;12:264–6.

[85] Burck PJ, Thakkare AL, Zimmerman RE. Antifertility action of sterol sulphate in the rabbit. J Reprod Fertil 1982;66:109–12.

[86] Malini T. Effects of β-sitosterol on reproductive tissues of male and female albino rats [doctoral thesis]. India: University of Madras.

[87] Malini T, Vanithakumari G. Antifertility effects of β-sitosterol in male albino rats. J Ethnopharmacol 1991;35(2):149–53.

[88] Jonas WB, Levin JS, editors. Essentials of complementary and alternative medicine. Philadelphia: Lippincott Williams & Wilkins; 1999.

[89] Novey DW, editor. Clinician's complete reference to complementary & alternative medicine. St. Louis (MO): Mosby; 2000.

[90] Micozzi MS, Koop CE, editors. Fundamentals of complementary and alternative medicine. 2nd edition. New York: Churchill Livingstone; 2001.
[91] Furnham A, Forey J. The attitudes, behaviors and beliefs of patients of conventional vs complementary (alternative) medicine. J Clin Psychol 1994;50:458–69.
[92] Astin JA. Why patients use alternative medicine. JAMA 1998;279:1548–53.
[93] Chez RA, Jonas WB, Eisenberg D. The physician and complementary and alternative medicine. In: Jonas WB, Levin JS, editors. Essentials of complementary and alternative medicine. Philadelphia: Lippincott Williams & Wilkins; 1999. p. 31–45.

Further readings

Blumenthal M, Busse WR, Goldberg A, et al. The complete German Commission E monographs: therapeutic guide to herbal medicines. Boston: American Botanical Council; 1998.

Brinker F. Herb contraindications and drug interactions. Sandy (OR): Eclectic Medical Publications; 2001.

Hudson T. Women's encyclopedia of natural medicine. Lincolnwood (IL): Keats Publishing; 1999.

Kass-Annese B, Danzed H. Natural birth control made simple. Alameda (CA): Hunter House; 2003.

McGuffin M, Hobbs C, Upton R, et al, editors. Botanical safety handbook. New York: CRC Press; 1997.

Murray M, Pizzorno J. Encyclopedia of natural medicine. Roseville (CA): Prima Publishing; 1998.

Riddle J. Eve's herbs. Cambridge (MA): Harvard University Press; 1997.

Schulz V, Hansel R, Blumenthal M, et al. Rational phytotherapy. Heidelberg (Germany): Springer–Verlag; 2004.

Tyler V. The honest herbal. New York: Pharmceutical Products Press; 1993.

Wechsler T. Taking charge of your fertility. New York: Harper Collins; 2002.

www.consumerlab.com.

www.herbalgram.com.

www.naturaldatabase.com.

www.naturesherbal.com.

www.sisterzeus.com.

ELSEVIER
SAUNDERS

ADOLESCENT
MEDICINE
CLINICS

Adolesc Med 16 (2005) 617–633

Current Contraceptive Research and Development

Kathleen Z. Reape, MD, FACOG

*Clinical Operations, Duramed Research, Inc., a subsidiary of Barr Pharmaceuticals, Inc.,
One Belmont Avenue, Suite 1100, Bala Cynwyd, PA 19004, USA*

Since the first oral contraceptive, norethynodrel, was approved in 1960, advances in contraceptive development and research have resulted in improved products and an expansion of the contraceptive options available to women. For oral contraceptive formulations, the marked decreases in estrogen and progestin content over the past 40 years have improved the safety of modern birth control pills by decreasing the risk of cardiovascular and thromboembolic adverse events. Other recent developments in contraceptive technology have included the introduction of new synthetic progestins, novel delivery systems and dosing regimens, and an increased focus on the noncontraceptive benefits of various contraceptive methods.

It is important that the level of contraceptive research be maintained or expanded and that new products continue to be brought to market. It is known that in terms of contraception, one size does not fit all. Women respond differently to combined oral contraceptive formulations; some will do well on a particular progestin, while others may have intolerable adverse effects. There is a need for a wide variety of contraceptive options. The average age of menarche in the United States is approximately 12 years, and the average age of menopause is approximately 51 years [1]. Modern trends toward delayed childbearing, decreased parity, and decreased duration of lactation mean that many women may require some method of contraception for 30 years or more, and the particular method or formulation that may be optimal or preferred for a woman at the age of 18 may be different than the method she chooses to use or can medically use at the age of 40. The choice of a contraceptive method is influenced not only by a woman's medical history, but also by her current social or family situation,

---

E-mail address: kreape@barrlabs.com

adolescent.theclinics.com

frequency of intercourse, desire for children and spacing of pregnancies, fecundity, preferred dosing frequency, level of effectiveness, noncontraceptive benefits, and cost of the method. Because of these influencing factors that vary throughout a woman's reproductive life, it is crucial that women have access to numerous safe and effective contraceptive options.

Recent and future trends in contraception

In the early to mid-1990s, there were few new contraceptive product approvals. In the past several years, however, new products have included low-dose estrogen-containing oral contraceptives (OCs), an OC formulated with a novel progestin, acne indications for selected combined OCs, a combined monthly hormonal injection, a long-lasting progestin-containing intrauterine device, a contraceptive vaginal ring, a contraceptive patch, and an extended-cycle OC. Factors driving these trends probably include improved tolerability and adverse effect profiles, reversibility, ease of use, and the desire for less frequent dosing and fewer withdrawal bleeding episodes, with the maintenance of high levels of efficacy. These recent trends in contraceptive research (changes in dosing regimen, variations in dose, introduction of novel progestins or estrogens, evaluation of noncontraceptive indications, and emergence of new delivery methods) are expected to continue in the future, and new products likely will reflect these trends.

Hormonal contraception

Hormonal methods of contraception include oral and nonoral products. The oral products are primarily combined oral contraceptives, but they also include progestin-only pills and emergency contraception. Nonoral contraceptive products include the transdermal patch, vaginal ring, injections, implants, and a hormone-releasing intrauterine system. Development of new hormonal products is focused on extended-cycle regimens, low-dose estrogen-containing products, the introduction of novel compounds, and the use of nonoral delivery systems (Box 1).

Oral hormonal contraceptive products

Extended cycle regimens
The first extended cycle oral contraceptive, levonorgestrel (LNG) 0.15 mg/ethinyl estradiol (EE) 0.03 mg tablets, was approved in 2003. It is a 91-day regimen consisting of 84 days of active tablets followed by 7 inactive tablets. This extended cycle regimen is designed to produce four withdrawal bleeding episodes per year, rather than the 13 episodes per year experienced with a conventional 28-day regimen. The incidence of breakthrough bleeding and spotting

Box 1. Categories of contraceptive products

Hormonal contraceptives

Oral products
Combination oral contraceptives

- Extended regimens
- Variations in hormone-free interval
- Low-dose
- Novel estrogens/progestins
- Noncontraceptive indications

Progestin-only contraceptives
Emergency contraception

Nonoral products
Transdermal delivery

- Patches
- Gels, creams, sprays

Vaginal rings
Injections
Implants
Hormone-releasing intrauterine devices (IUDs)
Male hormonal contraceptives

Nonhormonal contraceptives

Barrier methods

- Mechanical (condoms)
- Chemical (spermicides)

Nonhormonal IUDs
Dual protection: spermicide plus microbicide
Vaccines/immunocontraceptives
Sterilization

is increased on the extended regimen when compared with a conventional regimen, especially in the early extended cycles [2]. The 28-day oral contraceptive regimen (21 days of active tablets followed by 7 days of placebo tablets) that has been used for over 40 years was not based on scientific principle or medical necessity, but rather was designed to make the pill more acceptable to women by mimicking a natural 28-day menstrual cycle and providing reassurance each month that pregnancy had not occurred [3].

Other extended-cycle oral contraceptive regimens are in development. Seasonale Lo (LNG 0.10 mg/EE 0.02 mg tablets) is the same 91-day regimen as Seasonale (84 active tablets followed by 7 days of placebo) but contains lower doses of estrogen and progestin. The new drug application (NDA) for Seasonale Lo is expected to be filed this year.

Sulak [4,5] has shown that approximately 30% to 40% of women experience hormone-related withdrawal symptoms (such as nausea/vomiting, breast tenderness, pelvic pain, bloating/swelling) during the pill-free interval while using 28-day OCs, and symptomatic women may benefit from extending the number of active pills in a cycle. Additionally, continuous administration of active combined pills or modification of the usual hormone-free interval with the addition of low doses of ethinyl estradiol alone has been shown to result in less ovarian follicular activity than a 21/7 regimen (21 active followed by 7 placebo tablets per 28-day cycle), suggesting improved ovulation inhibition [6].

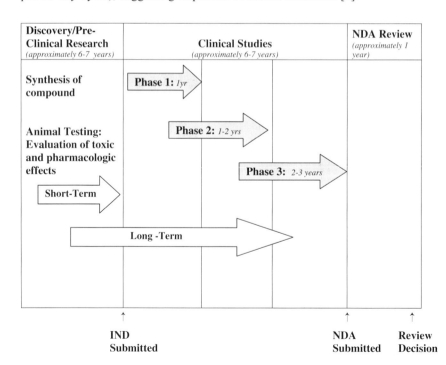

Fig. 1. New drug development process.

Another extended cycle regimen in development is levonorgestrel (LNG) (0.150 mg) and ethinyl estradiol (EE) (0.03 mg) and is administered for 84 days followed by 7 days of 10 μg of EE alone. The NDA was filed in the fall of 2004 [7] (Fig. 1, Table 1).

Levonorgestrel/ethinyl estradiol tablets containing 0.1 mg LNG and 0.02 mg EE are being developed as a continuous OC; that is, there are no regularly scheduled placebo intervals. It is designed to be administered daily for up to 1 year, which should result in inhibition of menses. Large clinical trials are ongoing to evaluate the safety and efficacy of Librel for preventing pregnancy in addition to its effects on premenstrual syndrome (PMS)/premenstrual dysphoric disorder (PMDD), acne, and cycle-related symptoms such as dysmenorrhea, irritability, and emotional lability. This product is projected to be available within the next year [8,9].

Researchers are working on another extended regimen oral contraceptive product using EE and drospirenone [10], but no further information is available, and the timing of the availability of this product is unknown.

Although not currently approved as extended use forms, other monthly contraceptive hormonal products would appear to be suitable for use in extended regimens. The NuvaRing (etonogestrel/EE vaginal ring) is being evaluated for 6 and 12 weeks and 12 months of use [11]. The OrthoEvra patch (norelgestromin/EE transdermal system) could be used in extended regimens by simply eliminating the placebo week and applying a patch instead. No published information is available regarding development of the OrthoEvra patch for extended use, however, so the status of this product is unknown.

Table 1
New drug development process

Step	Description
Preclinical research	Evaluation of drug's toxic and pharmacologic effects through in vitro and in vivo laboratory animal testing
IND	Investigational new drug—filed prior to initiating clinical trials in people
Phase 1	Initial studies of investigational drug in people, usually in healthy volunteers, to determine metabolic and pharmaologic actions and adverse effects with increasing doses, pharmacokinetic studies. Usually involves approximately 20–80 people.
Phase 2	Early controlled clinical studies to obtain preliminary data on effectiveness and short-term adverse effects in patients with the diesase or condition. May aid in identifying effective dosage. Usually involves 100 or more people.
Phase 3	Large clinical trials to determine effectiveness and safety; usually involves several hundred to several thousand people
NDA	New drug application: vehicle through which drug sponsors formally propose that the FDA approve a new pharmaceutical for sale in the United States. Information, data, and analyses provided by the sponsor in the NDA permit FDA reviewers to determine whether drug is safe and effective, whether labeling is appropriate, and whether manufacturing and quality controls are adequate.

Adapted from The new drug approval process. Available at: www.fda.gov/cder/handbook/develop. htm. Accessed November 2, 2004.

Extended regimens may be appealing to adolescents, particularly those who may prefer the convenience of fewer scheduled withdrawal bleeding episodes or the absence of bleeding altogether. When starting an extended regimen, adolescents should be counseled about the potential for increased breakthrough bleeding and spotting, particularly in the early cycles.

Low-dose formulations

The past 40 years of contraceptive development have resulted in marked decreases in the steroid content of modern combined oral contraceptives. Earlier pills routinely contained daily doses of 50 to 100 μg of estrogen and similarly high doses of progestins. Today, most marketed oral contraceptives contain only 20 to 35 μg of estrogen, which has decreased the incidence of major (eg, cardiovascular and venous thromboembolic events) and minor (eg, nausea or swelling) adverse events without compromising contraceptive efficacy [3].

The trend toward lower-dose regimens continues. Yaz (drospirenone and EE tablets 3.0 mg/0.020 mg), which is given in a 24-day active and 4-day placebo regimen, received an approvable letter in November 2004. An approvable letter indicates that the Food and Drug Administration (FDA) generally approves of the application but that more data are required. Pharmaceutical researchers hope to have Yaz approved this year. The currently marketed in drospirenone and EE tablets 3.0mg/0.030 mg oral contraceptive contains a higher dose of EE and is administered in a 21-day active/7-day placebo regimen [10].

Levonorgestrel/ethinyl estradiol tablets, a continuous regimen, and levonorgestrel/ethinyl estradiol (0.10 mg/0.02 mg) tablets, an extended cycle regimen both contain a daily 20 μg dose of EE. With extended or continuous regimens and fewer placebo tablets, the additional weeks of estrogen exposure may pose a theoretical increased risk of thromboembolic events, but studies have not demonstrated this [12].

Adolescents may find low-dose (20 μg EE) oral contraceptives easier to tolerate, with the potential for fewer steroid-related adverse effects (eg, nausea, bloating, or breast tenderness) than formulations containing higher doses of estrogen. Cycle control for new low-dose formulations must be acceptable, however, or dissatisfaction and method discontinuation may occur. Additionally, data are somewhat limited, but the potential exists for adverse effects of low-dose oral contraceptives on bone growth and attainment of peak bone mass in adolescents, and this should be considered when assessing contraceptive options.

Novel compounds—progestins and estrogens

Even though there are numerous synthetic progestins available and marketed in current combination oral contraceptives, new progestins are being developed. Progestins may have estrogenic, androgenic, glucocorticoid, and mineralocorticoid effects in addition to their progestational activity. No available synthetic progestin exactly replicates the properties of natural progesterone. Natural progesterone (produced by the ovaries) is metabolized rapidly and cannot be given orally in high enough doses for contraception, so the search for a similar synthetic progestin continues. Most currently available oral contraceptive progestins are derivatives of 19 nor-testosterone and therefore have the potential for androgenic adverse effects [13]. Drospirenone is a 17-α-spirolactone derivative and is in its own class as a progestin. Because it is a spironolactone analog, it may possess certain properties, such as diuretic effects, that make it unique as a progestin.

The progestin trimegestone is being developed for use in oral contraception [7]. Trimegestone is a 19-norprogesterone derivative and may have less androgenic adverse effects than other synthetic progestins. It is highly potent and has a pharmacologic profile similar to progesterone [13]. Trimegestone is available and marketed for use as hormone therapy in Europe.

Several new methods are being developed using the progestin compound (16-methylene-17α-acetoxy-19-nor-pregn-4-ene-3, 20 dione). Like trimegestone, Nestorone is a 19-norporgesterone derivative and is similar to natural progesterone. It is not active orally, and research has included studies on a single rod Nestorone implant, some form of transdermal delivery system, and a 1-year combination vaginal ring (Nestorone and EE) [14].

A novel category of compounds includes the antiprogestins (progesterone antagonists) and selective progesterone receptor modulators or SPRMs. Most of these compounds are at an early point in the development process, so it is unlikely that products will be available in the near future. Because progesterone plays such an intrinsic role in the reproductive cycle, antiprogestins have great potential as regulators of reproduction. They can suppress ovulation and alter endometrial development, making them suitable for contraception [15]. This category of compounds also has the potential for use as estrogen-free contraceptive products. Long-term safety and effectiveness of these compounds, and comparison to currently available methods will need to be evaluated.

A nonsteroidal antiprogestin, tanaproget, is being developed for use in contraception, and phase III trials started in late 2004. Tanaproget is being developed alone as the first nonsteroidal oral contraceptive, and it is being developed in combination with EE as a combination oral contraceptive. It is anticipated that the tanaproget alone product will be available in early 2008, with the combination product available in late 2008 [8].

Org 33,628, a progestin/antiprogestin combination, is being developed for contraception. Phase II trials are in progress [16,17].

An antiprogestin molecule, CDB-2914, is being evaluated for use in a contraceptive ring and intrauterine system. This molecule has potential to be used as a continuous contraceptive, resulting in amenorrhea. An investigational new drug (IND) application for a clinical study of a ring releasing CDB-2914 was submitted to the FDA, and a phase I trial was conducted in Chile and the Dominican Republic. Use of this compound in an intrauterine system is in the preclinical phase [14].

Ethinyl estradiol has been the primary synthetic estrogen used in oral contraceptives for decades, and it is very potent when given orally. 17-β-estradiol is the most potent natural estrogen and is the major estrogen secreted by the ovaries. It is relatively inactive when administered orally, however. It has been postulated that a combined oral contraceptive with 17β-estradiol might produce fewer adverse effects on the hemostatic system than those containing EE [1]. Attempts at developing hormonal contraceptives using estradiol have not been very successful because of high rates of irregular bleeding and difficulties in maintaining sufficient blood levels for ovulation inhibition because of rapid metabolism of the orally administered compound. In 1996, Csemiczky described a regimen using 3 mg of micronized estradiol in combination with desogestrel and evaluated ovarian function, bleeding patterns, and estradiol levels for three treatment cycles [18].

Schering AG has an oral contraceptive pill in phase III development that contains estradiol and the progestin dienogest. This is designed to provide contraception for women in the late reproductive years (ages 35 to 50 years) and is being evaluated for potential beneficial effects on dysfunctional uterine bleeding [10].

Nonoral hormonal products

Transdermal delivery systems

Partly because of the success of the OrthoEvra patch, other transdermal delivery systems for contraception are in various stages of development. There are advantages, particularly in the adolescent population, to less frequent dosing, and there may be potential benefits in terms of adverse effect profile, as a result of eliminating the hepatic first pass effects with transdermal delivery. New trends in transdermal delivery may include extended cycle regimens using patches, multiple colors and sizes of patches, and other nonpatch methods of transdermal delivery, such as creams, gels, and sprays.

Three different 7-day transdermal contraceptive patches containing EE and LNG are in phase II clinical testing. The patch in development by Agile is constructed of translucent material and is virtually invisible once the patch is applied to the skin [19]. This patch would be applied weekly in a 3 weeks on, 1 week off regimen.

An estrogen/progestin patch for fertility control (FC Patch, containing the progestin gestodene and EE), which is applied once a week, is being evaluated. This product is currently in phase III clinical trials [10,16].

Early clinical work has been done on the progestin, Nestorone, delivered by means of a transdermal gel, but no further information is available on this product [14].

Contraceptive rings

Etonogestrel/ethinyl estradiol vaginal ring was the first vaginal ring approved for contraception, in 2001. It contains etonogestrel as the progestin, and EE. It is designed to be placed in the vagina continuously for 3 weeks of each cycle. The ring is removed for 1 week, allowing for a withdrawal bleeding episode.

The vaginal ring is discreet and allows for less frequent dosing than either oral or transdermal delivery, and, as is the case with transdermal administration, there is no hepatic first pass effect. Unlike implants, rings are user-controlled, and do not require clinician insertion or removal. Hormones are released continuously from the ring, so lower doses of estrogen and progestin are required. NuvaRing releases 120 µg/d of etonogestrel (a metabolite of desogestrel) and 15 µg/d of EE. Lower serum concentrations of estrogen are obtained with NuvaRing than with oral or transdermal products, potentially resulting in a low incidence of hormone-related adverse effects. NuvaRing has been shown to be highly effective, with excellent cycle control [20]. A large international study of 1950 women demonstrated a high level of user and partner acceptability for the contraceptive ring [21].

There are fewer contraceptive ring products in development than either oral or transdermal products, perhaps because of the specialized technology and manufacturing requirements and smaller size of the marketplace. Ring technology seems particularly suited for extended regimen use. A large, open-label randomized, multi-center trial of continuous regimens with NuvaRing is ongoing. Subjects are randomized to either the approved regimen; 6 weeks of continuous use followed by a 1-week ring-free period; 12 weeks of continuous use followed by a 1-week ring-free period; or 12 months of continuous use without any ring-free periods, to induce amenorrhea [11]. It appears likely that in the future, NuvaRing will be available for use in an extended regimen.

Several variations of vaginal rings, employing different hormonal combinations are being evaluated, and new molecules are being tested for use in vaginal rings. A 1-year combination ring containing Nestorone (150 µg/d) and EE (15 µg/d) has completed phase II development, and plans for phase III are underway. The ring would be inserted for 3 weeks, then removed for 1 week, allowing for a withdrawal bleeding episode. The ring is designed to contain sufficient quantities of the hormones to provide contraception for a full year, following the 3-weeks-in, 1-week-out schedule. A Nestorone-only vaginal ring to be used for up to 12 months in lactating women also is being evaluated, and a natural progesterone ring is distributed in Chile and Peru for use in the same population. As noted previously the novel antiprogestin molecule CDB-2914 also is being evaluated for use in a contraceptive ring [14].

Because of the user autonomy, potential for decreased adverse effects, and less frequent dosing, vaginal rings are an appropriate contraceptive option for adolescents. Initial resistance to the concept of transvaginal delivery may be overcome with education, instruction, and counseling. Providing reassurance of user and partner satisfaction and comfort also may be helpful to adolescents considering this method.

Injections

Two phase III multi-center 1-year studies were performed to assess the efficacy, safety, and subject satisfaction of a low-dose subcutaneous formulation of depot medroxyprogesterone acetate (DMPA-SC) [22]. Compared with the currently marketed intramuscular Depo-Provera contraceptive injection (medroxyprogesterone acetate injectable suspension), which contains 150 mg of MPA, the subcutaneous depot contains 104 mg of MPA. Both are administered every 3 months. In the trials, the subcutaneous formulation was shown to be highly efficacious and well tolerated. The NDA for subcutaneous Depo-Provera was submitted to the FDA in June 2003 and depo-subQ provera 104 (medroxyprogesterone acetate injectable suspension 104 mg/0.65 mL) was approved in December, 2004. Subcutaneous injections may be less painful than intramuscular injections, and the potential for self-administration may aid in compliance, particularly among adolescents, since many may have difficulty in physically getting to see a clinician every 3 months for an injection.

As long-acting progestin-only products, the DMPA injections offer estrogen-free contraception without the need for frequent dosing. Prolonged use of DMPA may lead to a decrease in bone mineral density, which may not be completely reversible; the potential impact on bone mineral density should be considered when assessing DMPA as a contraceptive option. A common effect is irregular menstrual bleeding, which decreases with time, usually resulting in amenorrhea. In some users, there also may be a delay in return to fertility. For adolescents, this may not be an issue, although a false sense of contraceptive security should be avoided. If injections are discontinued and pregnancy is not desired, another method of birth control should be initiated immediately.

Implants

The single-rod contraceptive implant, Implanon, contains the progestin etonogestrel and has an average release rate of 40 µg per day. It is a single flexible 1 inch rod inserted under the skin of the upper arm, and it provides contraception for 3 years. This is a non-estrogen–containing product and may be used by women who cannot tolerate or have contraindications to estrogens. Insertion and removal must be performed by a clinician, but it is simpler than with the six-rod Norplant product, since only one rod is placed. The FDA had granted Implanon approvable status in 2004. It is expected that Implanon may be available in the United States this year. It has been available in Europe since 1999 [17].

A two-rod contraceptive implant system, Jadelle, releases the progestin, LNG, and is FDA-approved for 5 years of continuous use. This product has not yet been marketed in the United States. A single rod, Nestorone-releasing implant also is being developed [14]. In a 2-year clinical trial of 300 women in Latin America, the Nestorone implant was shown to be effective, and further work is being done [23]. It is not known if or when either Jadelle or the Nestorone implant will be available in the United States.

Subdermal implants may be appealing to adolescents who desire highly effective, long-term, reversible contraception. Insertion and removal require a trained clinician, and there have been complications reported with both insertions and removals. Once the implant has been placed, there is no effort required on the part of the user. Because implants contain only a progestin, these products are suitable for women who cannot tolerate or have contraindications to estrogens.

Noncontraceptive indications

An emerging trend in contraceptive research is the pursuit of noncontraceptive indications, particularly among oral contraceptive products. Norgestimate/ethinyl estradiol tablets changed the contraceptive landscape in 1997 when it received the indication for the treatment of moderate-to-severe acne. Direct-to-consumer marketing brought women to the clinician's office, requesting a specific oral contraceptive; consequently, in a short period of time, OrthoTri-Cyclen became known as the acne pill. The demonstration of a statistically and clinically significant effect in a clinical trial and approval for a specific indication allow for incorporation of that information into the product promotional material, leading to potential differentiation of the product and user-driven requests for a particular brand. Additionally, because all women are different, additional data on various conditions may help clinicians narrow the range of products and more clearly define the contraceptive options for an individual user, resulting in a positive user experience, potentially increased adherence, and fewer unintended pregnancies.

Since the approval of norgestimate/ethinyl estradiol tablets for acne, other products have conducted acne clinical trials. Norethindrone acetate and ethinyl estradiol tablets also received the indication for treating moderate-to-severe acne.

Premenstrual syndrome and PMDD also have been studied in contraceptive users. PMS/PMDD and acne trials are ongoing with Yaz. Librel also is being evaluated for use in treating symptoms of PMS/PMDD [9,10].

For certain adolescents, some of these symptoms may be particularly troublesome. Data from these trials may assist in selecting an appropriate contraceptive for an individual, and if an adolescent notices improvements in acne, dysmenorrhea, or premenstrual symptoms, she is probably more likely to be satisfied with and adherent to her contraceptive regimen.

Emergency contraception

Every sexually active adolescent should be aware of the existence of emergency contraception. This is not a substitute for a primary means of contraception, because more effective methods are available. Rather, emergency contraception is intended as a method of preventing pregnancy after an episode of unprotected intercourse or in the case of contraceptive accident. It should be considered in cases of sexual assault, when condoms break, or with a lapse in the use of a primary method. Treatment needs to be started as soon as possible and within 120 hours after unprotected intercourse, because efficacy decreases as the interval between intercourse and initiation of treatment increases [24]. Current product labeling states that use should be initiated within 72 hours of unprotected intercourse, but good efficacy has been demonstrated with an interval as long as 120 hours [24,25].

Yuzpe described a method of emergency contraception using conventional combination oral contraceptives [3]. Levonorgestrel and ethinyl estradiol tablets, a combination product containing 0.25 mg LNG and 0.5 mg EE, was approved in 1998 specifically for emergency contraception, however, because of nausea and vomiting from the high estrogen content, this product is no longer produced. Levonorgestrel tablets (0.75 mg) was the second product approved specifically for emergency contraception, in 1999. It contains only LNG, reducing the adverse effects and risks associated with high-dose estrogen administration.

In 2003, a supplemental new drug application (sNDA) was submitted for an over-the-counter (OTC) Plan B product. In May 2004, the company received a not approvable letter for this application, stating that it did "not provide adequate data to support a conclusion that Plan B can be used safely by young adolescent women for emergency contraception without the professional supervision of a (licensed) practitioner." The manufacturer is continuing to pursue over-the-counter status for Plan B [24]. Access and awareness remain significant barriers to the use of emergency contraception that need to be addressed.

Male hormonal contraception

Current choices available to men for contraception are limited and (with the exception of vasectomy) of variable efficacy. For adolescent males, there are condoms and less satisfactory options such as abstinence and withdrawal. It is important to counsel both male and female adolescents that none of the birth control methods discussed previously provides protection against sexually transmitted infections (STIs). Condoms play a pivotal role in decreasing the risk of transmission of infections, and this needs to be emphasized.

From a scientific standpoint, development of male hormonal contraceptives is an interesting and challenging area of research. There are, however, significant barriers that might preclude such a product from reaching the market. First and foremost, there are safety and efficacy concerns. Hormonal contraception in men is complex, with the goal being reversible cessation of sperm production without compromising libido. Large doses of testosterone produce azoospermia, but they also may produce significant adverse effects, including prostate enlargement. Current research is focused on lower doses of androgens (to diminish adverse effects) in combination with progestins or gonadotropin releasing hormone (GNRH) antagonists. Various androgen/progestin combinations have been studied and have been shown to induce azoospermia and clinically significant oligospermia more quickly than androgens alone, although the numbers of patients in these studies are relatively small [26,27]. A progestin/androgen combination is undergoing phase II trials for male contraception [17]. There is no convenient formulation of androgen; most are delivered by means of implant or frequent injection because of the pharmacokinetic profiles of the available preparations.

Recently, a long-acting preparation, testosterone undecanoate (TU), has been studied and may be a promising candidate for use as a male hormonal contraceptive. A multi-center, phase II trial in 308 Chinese men using a loading dose of 1000 mg followed by monthly intramuscular injections of 500 mg demonstrated azoospermia in 98% of subjects [28]. Schering AG is pursuing development of this compound, and it is in phase III clinical trials [10,16].

Male hormonal methods are being developed using MENT (7α-methyl-19-nortestosterone), a synthetic steroid that is similar to testosterone. A MENT implant has been studied in a 1-year dose finding trial, and other studies that combine MENT implants with a synthetic progestin are underway. Delivery of MENT may be accomplished transdermally; use in transdermal gels and patches is being evaluated [14].

In addition to the complexity of the hormonal regimens, other potential barriers to the use of male hormonal contraception include the delay between the initiation of treatment and the onset of the contraceptive effect. The mechanism of action is the inhibition of spermatogenesis, meaning that additional contraception would be required for approximately 3 months. Return to fertility could be delayed also. The cost of a male hormonal contraceptive may be significantly higher compared with the cost of condoms and female methods of birth control. There may be poor acceptance among men to the concept of male contraception and a lack of trust among women regarding male fertility control. Male hormonal contraception will not offer any protection against STIs. Long-term safety, efficacy, and reversibility data will need to be available, and this method is likely to be most appealing to couples in stable, monogamous relationships as a reversible alternative to vasectomy.

Nonhormonal contraception

Nonhormonal methods of contraception available in the United States include copper-releasing IUDs, barrier methods (mechanical male and female condoms, diaphragms, chemical-spermicides), dual methods that combine an intravaginal spermicide with a microbicide to prevent pregnancy and STIs, and vaccines, and sterilization. IUDs are generally not recommended for adolescents, and sterilization is not an option. Compared with other available methods, diaphragms and other female barrier devices have a relatively high contraceptive failure rate and are not routinely used in the adolescent population.

Microbicides/spermicides

Microbicides with spermicidal activity, in theory, offer significant advantages over existing methods because of their dual action of preventing pregnancy and infection, but there is some concern about the level of contraceptive efficacy.

Table 2
New contraceptive products in development

Product/compound	Company	Status	Comments
Oral contraceptives			
Yaz	Schering AG	Approvable 11/04	24/4 Regimen; 3 mg drospirenone/20 EE
Seasonique	Duramed	NDA filed-10/04	91-day extended regimen; 84 days of 150 LNG/30 EE followed by 7 days of 10 EE
Seasonale Lo	Duramed	Phase III completed	84/7 regimen; 100 LNG/20 EE
Dienogest/estradiol	Schering AG	Phase III	Use in 35–50-year-olds, Dysfunctional uterine bleeding
Librel	Wyeth	Phase III	Continuous use up to 1 year (100 LNG/20 EE); PMS/PMDD symptoms, acne
ORG 33628	Organon	Phase II	Antiprogestin; estrogen-free contraception
Tanaproget	Wyeth	Phase II	Nonsteroidal antiprogestin
Trimegestone/EE	Duramed	Phase II	
Tanaproget/EE combination	Wyeth	Phase I	
Yasmin extended cycle	Schering AG	?	
Nonoral hormonal contraceptives–transdermal			
FC Patch; Gestodene/EE	Schering AG	Phase III	Weekly patch
7-day Patch; LNG/EE	Agile Therapeutics	Phase II	Translucent patch
Nestorone	Population Council	Phase I	Gel, patch; combination with estradiol
Non-Oral Hormonal Contraceptives–Vaginal Rings			
Progesterone ring	Population Council	Approved in Chile, Peru	Contraception for lactating women

Name	Sponsor	Status	Description
NuvaRing extended use	Organon	Phase III	6 or 12 weeks, 12 months duration of use
Nestorone/EE ring	Population Council	Phase II completed	Monthly administration (3 wks in, 1 wk out); use for 1 year
CDB 2914	Population Council	Phase I	Antiprogestin; also evaluating for use in IUD
Nestorone ring	Population Council	?	Use for up to 12 months; lactating women
Injections/implants			
Jadelle	Population Council	Approved	2 rod levonorgestrel implant; approved for 5 years of use
Implanon	Organon	Approvable 11/04	1 rod etonorgestrel implant; 3 years of use
depo-subQ provera 104	Pfizer	Approved	
Nestorone implant	Population Council	Phase II	1 rod implant
Male hormonal contraceptives			
Testosterone undeconoate	Schering AG	Phase III	Monthly intramuscular injections
MENT	Population Council	Phase II	7-alpha-mehtyl-19-nortestosterone implants
Progestin/androgen combination	Organon	Phase II	
Other—microbicides, spermicides, vaccines			
Carraguard	Population Council	Phase III	Microbicidal gel to decrease male to female transmission of HIV; noncontraceptive
PRO 2000 gel	Indevus	Phase I	Contraceptive microbicide

To avoid having to use two methods of birth control to prevent infection and pregnancy, contraceptive efficacy of a combined spermicide/microbicide should be similar to that of currently available hormonal contraceptives. Much of the research and development in this area have been done by biotechnology firms and not-for-profit organizations [27]. A large-scale randomized, double blind, placebo-controlled trial is being conducted in South Africa of the microbicidal carrageenan gel. The trial began in March 2004. The primary objectives of this trial are "to determine the efficacy of Carraguard gel in preventing male-to-female transmission of HIV when applied before vaginal sex, and to evaluate its safety when used for up to 2 years." The goal is to enroll over 6000 women in the study [14].

PRO 2000 topical microbicide contraceptive gel is under development and is currently in phase II clinical trials to evaluate its use for preventing pregnancy and STIs, including HIV, herpes simplex virus, *Chlamydia trachomatis,* and *Neisseria gonorrhoeae* [16,27].

Contraceptive vaccines

Contraceptive vaccines have been of interest to the research community for some time. There remain doubts about safety, however, specifically the potential for long-term effects on fertility and antibody formation that could interfere with other hormonal functions. Additionally, there is concern about the possibility of administration without consent. A few vaccines that target human chorionic gonadotropin have been evaluated in early-stage trials, but no further information is available, and it appears that much of the research activity related to these compounds essentially has been discontinued.

These nonhormonal methods, with the exception of condoms, are not available yet or are generally not appropriate for use in adolescents. Research on contraceptive vaccines, microbicides, dual protection methods, and male hormonal methods is still in the early stages, and questions about safety and efficacy, particularly in the adolescent population, remain to be answered.

Summary

Numerous recent new product approvals in the field of contraception have resulted in the expansion of options available to women and increased interest in reproductive research. It is important to have a variety of safe and effective contraceptive formulations, methods, and delivery options available to men and women, so it is imperative that contraceptive research and development continue, both in the public and private sectors. Despite challenges in this field, ongoing research and development activity for oral and nonoral hormonal contraceptive products and nonhormonal methods is quite robust, (Table 2) and should ensure that new products continue to become available.

References

[1] Speroff L, Glass R, Kase N. Clinical gynecologic endocrinology and infertility. 6th edition. Baltimore (MD): Lippincott Williams & Wilkins; 1999.

[2] Anderson F, Hait H. A multi-center, randomized study of an extended cycle oral contraceptive. Contraception 2003;68(2):89–96.

[3] Speroff L, Darney P. A clinical guide for contraception. 2nd edition. Baltimore (MD): Williams & Wilkins; 1996.

[4] Sulak P, Scow R, Preece C, et al. Hormone withdrawal symptoms in oral contraceptive users. Obstet Gynecol 2000;95(2):261–6.

[5] Sulak P, Cressman B, Waldrop E, et al. Extending the duration of active oral contraceptive pills to manage hormone withdrawal symptoms. Obstet Gynecol 1997;89(2):179–83.

[6] Schlaff W, Lynch A, Hughes H, et al. Manipulation of the pill-free interval in oral contraceptive pill users: the effect on follicular suppression. Am J Obstet Gynecol 2004;190(4):943–51.

[7] Investor relations. Available at: http://www.barrlabs.com/home.html. Accessed November 10, 2004.

[8] Dey M, Constantine G. Wyeth: the leader in women's health—yesterday, today, and tomorrow. Sexuality. Reproduction & Menopause 2004;2(3):181–4.

[9] Investor Relations. Wyeth analyst meeting, June 2, 2004. Emerging commercial candidates. Available at: http://www.wyeth.com/index.asp. Accessed November 10, 2004.

[10] Research and Development. Available at: http://www.schering.de. Accessed November 10, 2004.

[11] Aarts J, Miller L. Design of an open-label, randomized trial of continuous regimens with NuvaRing. Obstet Gynecol 2003;101(4):14S.

[12] US prescribing information. Seasonale. Revised September 2003.

[13] Sitruk-Ware R. Progestogens in hormonal replacement therapy: new molecules, risks, and benefits. Menopause 2002;9(1):6–15.

[14] Biomedicine. Product development. Available at: http://www.popcouncil.org. Accessed November 11, 2004.

[15] Spitz IM, Croxatto H, Robbins A. Antiprogestins: mechanisms of action and contraceptive potential. Annu Rev Pharmacol Toxicol 1996;36:47–81.

[16] From pipeline to market. R&D Directions 2004;10(6):35–74.

[17] Drug development. Available at: http://www.organon.com. Accessed November 11, 2004.

[18] Csemiczky G, Dieben T, Bennink H, et al. The pharmacodynamic effects of an oral contraceptive containing 3 mg micronized 17-β estradiol and 0.150 mg desogestrel for 21 days, followed by 0.030 mg desogestrel only for 7 days. Contraception 1996;54:333–8.

[19] Press releases. Available at: http://agiletherapeutics.com. Accessed November 11, 2004.

[20] Dieben T, Roumen F, Apter D. Efficacy, cycle control and user acceptability of a novel combined contraceptive vaginal ring. Obstet Gynecol 2002;100:585–93.

[21] Novak A, de la Loge C, Abetz L, et al. The combined contraceptive vaginal ring, NuvaRing: an international study of user acceptability. Contraception 2003;67(3):187–94.

[22] Darney P, Jain J, Jakimiuk A. Zero pregnancies with new low-dose depot medroxyprogesterone acetate subcutaneous injection for contraception. Fertil Steril 2004;82(Suppl 2):S105.

[23] Sivin I, Croxatto H, Bahamondes L, et al. Two-year performance of a Nestorone-releasing contraceptive implant: a three-center study of 300 women. Contraception 2004;69(2):137–44.

[24] About Plan B. Available at: http://go2planb.com. Accessed November 11, 2004.

[25] Von Hertzen H, Piaggio G, Ding J, et al. Low dose mifepristone and two regimens of levonorgestrel for emergency contraception: a WHO multi-centre randomised trial. Lancet 2002;360:1803–10.

[26] Wang C, Swerdloff R. Male hormonal contraception. Am J Obstet Gynecol 2004;190:S60–8.

[27] Schwartz J, Gabelnick H. Current contraceptive research. Perspect Sex Reprod Health 2002;34(6):310–6.

[28] Gu Y, Wang X, Xu D, et al. A multi-center contraceptive efficacy study of injectable testosterone undecanoate in healthy Chinese men. J Clin Endocrinol Metab 2003;88:562–8.

ADOLESCENT
MEDICINE
CLINICS

ELSEVIER
SAUNDERS

Adolesc Med 16 (2005) 635–644

Contraceptive Choices for Chronically Ill Adolescents

Elissa B. Gittes, MD[a,b,c,*], Julie L. Strickland, MD, MPH[a,d]

[a]University of Missouri-Kansas City School of Medicine, 2411 Holmes, Kansas City, MO 64108, USA
[b]Children's Mercy Hospital, Development and Behavioral Sciences, 2401 Gillham Road,
Kansas City, MO 64108, USA
[c]Children's Mercy South, 5808 West 110th Street, Overland Park, KS 66211, USA
[d]Division of Gynecology, 2401 Gillham Road, Children's Mercy Hospital,
Kansas City, MO 64108, USA

All adolescents, including those with a disability or chronic medical condition, experience psychosocial and physiological changes during adolescence and have the need to be regarded as sexual beings.

Chronic illness affects about 10% of children and adolescents by the age of 18 [1]. Youth with disabilities experience the same psychosocial development as do their healthy peers. Adolescents with chronic illness have sexual interests that also parallel those of their healthy peers. A study from 1996 showed no differences between adolescents with and without disability in those ever having intercourse, age of sexual debut, or pregnancy [2]. Sexual behaviors in boys and girls with visible compared with nonvisible medical conditions showed no differences in sexual behavior [2]. This implies that physical disability does not interfere with sexuality and the social needs of the adolescent.

Because of stress or inadequate nutrition, physiological changes of puberty may be delayed in chronically ill adolescents; however, youth experiencing menses must be considered fertile and at risk for unwanted pregnancy. In fact, because of advances in medical care and knowledge of the disease process, adolescents with some previously early fatal illness are now surviving into adulthood. Pregnancy for some teenagers with chronic conditions can result in significant morbidity and mortality. Safe and effective forms of contraception

* Corresponding author. Children's Mercy South, 5808 West 110th Street, Overland Park, KS, 66211.

  E-mail address: egittes@cmh.edu (E.B. Gittes).

1547-3368/05/$ – see front matter. Published by Elsevier Inc.
doi:10.1016/j.admecli.2005.05.002

adolescent.theclinics.com

are available for chronically ill adolescents; however, the particular medical illness needs to be considered when selecting a method.

This article reviews some chronic medical conditions and offers various contraceptive options for the adolescent.

Neurological disorders

Headaches are common complaints in adolescents. They can be divided into vascular, or migraine, and nonvascular types. Nonvascular headaches, including tension or muscular contraction subtypes, have no alteration in prevalence or risk with the use of hormonal contraception.

A hypothetical link exists between estrogen and vascular, or migraine, headaches. It has been observed that migraine headaches can be precipitated by the onset of menses in susceptible women. In addition, for adolescents on low-dose oral contraceptive pills (OCPs), most migraines occurred while they were taking the placebo, hormone-free pills. Migraines associated with menses (catamenial headaches) seem to be related to the drop in estrogen levels during monthly menses. A clear association between uncomplicated migraine headaches and estrogen-containing contraception has not been established [3]. In adolescents with uncomplicated migraines, low-dose OCPs or the OrthoEvra patch may be considered.

For girls with migraine headaches with neurological symptoms, however, data are convincing that there is an association between estrogen and risk of cerebral ischemia. A large study at five European centers found a statistically significant increase in risk of ischemic stroke in women with migraines and neurological symptoms [4]. A study in the United States confirmed this finding, as women with complicated migraines on OCPs had a higher incidence of ischemic stroke compared with those not on OCPs [5]. Girls with complicated migraine headaches must avoid use of estrogen-containing contraception. Progesterone-only methods, such as Medroxyprogesterone acetate (DMPA), the Mirena intra-uterine device (IUD), or barrier methods, are options for these girls.

Epilepsy is a common problem in teenagers. Although there is not strong evidence for an association between estrogen/progestin contraception and exacerbation of seizures [6], an understanding of the risk of pregnancy in an adolescent with epilepsy is especially important. Certain antiepileptic drugs induce hepatic enzymes, which can decrease estrogen and progesterone concentrations, leading to irregular vaginal bleeding and higher risk of contraceptive failure [7]. This effect has been seen with the more common anticonvulsants phenobarbital, phenytoin, carbamazepine, felbamate, and topiramate. Valproate, gabapentin, lamotrigine, and tiagabine did not lower serum estrogen/progesterone levels; however, the doses of these four anticonvulsants used in clinical studies were lower than what typically is prescribed [8–15].

Pregnancy in a woman on antiepileptic medication can carry significant risk for the fetus, because various anticonvulsants are known teratogens [16].

Contraceptive recommendations include prescribing a high-dose combination OCP containing 50 μg ethinyl estradiol (EE) with a concurrent barrier method. DMPA has not been evaluated specifically regarding contraceptive efficacy in women on anticonvulsants; however, pregnancies in these women have not been reported [17]. Because DMPA may be beneficial in reducing seizure activity, this method would be a good contraceptive choice [18]. Other contraceptive options for adolescents with epilepsy include the Mirena IUD or barrier method alone.

Adolescents with other illnesses such as bipolar disorder, binge-eating disorder, or other psychiatric conditions for which anticonvulsants are prescribed require the same contraceptive considerations as described for epilepsy [19].

Endocrine disorders

Teenagers with thyroid disease or hyperprolactinemia can select from any of the available contraception methods without concern for adverse effects on their illness. For girls on levothyroxine for hypothyroidism, evaluating free T4 and thyrotropin (TSH) after completing two cycles of estrogen-containing contraception is advisable [19]. For girls with hyperprolactinemia in whom a diagnosis of pituitary adenoma is ruled out, estrogen-containing methods provide the additional benefits of restoring regular menses, preventing further bone loss, and providing effective pregnancy prevention.

In diabetics without hypertension, nephropathy, retinopathy, or peripheral vascular disease, data support the use of low-dose OCPs as safe and effective contraception [20]. In fact, the newer progestins (desogestrel, norgestimate, and gestodene) appear to affect carbohydrate metabolism less than some of the older progestins [21].

Estrogen-containing contraception is contraindicated in diabetics with peripheral vascular disease. DMPA is a safe option for pregnancy prevention. It also has less effect on lipids compared with OCPs [22]. Barrier methods are also effective, but they mandate motivation from the adolescent. Coordination of care by practitioners prescribing contraception and those managing the diabetes is optimal, as blood pressure, weight, and lipid status should be monitored.

Cardiac

Children born with congenital heart lesions are being managed effectively and are surviving into adulthood. Pregnancy and contraception need to be addressed, as various lesions with right-to-left shunting or left ventricular dysfunction carry a very high maternal mortality rate.

In adolescents with congenital heart disease, there is a significant risk of thromboembolism because of increased circulation of clotting factors by stimulating hepatic production of serum globulins. Thus, estrogen-containing contraception, such as OCPs or the OrthoEvra patch, should not be used by girls with coronary heart disease, congestive heart failure, cardiac shunts, or low output heart conditions [23]. Contraception containing only progesterone does not increase thrombosis risk and offers an alternative form of hormonal contraception for these girls. In girls who are candidates for DMPA also are being treated with anticoagulants for their heart lesion. The Mirena IUD or barrier contraception may be an option for a select group of girls with stable heart disease.

In adolescents with hypertension, once again the risks associated with pregnancy need to be weighed against those of the contraceptive method. OCPs lead to a small but definitive increase in blood pressure of 8 mm Hg systolic and 6 mm Hg diastolic readings [24]. A causal relationship from the slight elevation in blood pressure to increase risk of vascular complications has not been determined definitively. Investigations of the relationship between OCPs and risk of stroke or myocardial infarction in hypertensive women show conflicting results. A large World Health Care Organization (WHO) study in Europe found an increase in ischemic events in hypertensive women on OCPs, while two case-control studies in the United States showed no substantial increased risk [25–27]. It appears that the relative risk for hypertensive women on OCPs for heart ischemia or stroke is increased; however, the absolute risk remains low.

In nonsmoking, hypertensive girls desiring OCPs, low-dose preparations with 35 µg or less of EE may be prescribed if the blood pressure is well-controlled, and there is no end-organ damage. Close monitoring of blood pressure is necessary. If the blood pressure status remains stable on estrogen/progesterone combination contraception, OCP use can be continued. Other alternatives for adolescents with hypertension include DMPA, the Mirena IUD, and barrier methods.

Renal disease

Teenagers with a history of kidney disease in childhood, such as nephrotic syndrome, who are medically stable and without impaired renal function or hypertension, are good candidates for OCPs, the OrthoEvra patch, DMPA, the Mirena IUD, and barrier contraception methods. Although adolescents with chronic renal failure and compromised health status are often anovulatory and amenorrheic, adolescents on dialysis or with relatively stable renal status may ovulate and have normal menstruation. For these girls, contraception needs to be considered. Estrogen-containing methods should be avoided in a teenager with chronic renal failure and significant hypertension or risk of thrombo-embolism. A progesterone-only or barrier contraceptive is the hormonal method of choice. The progesterone-impregnated Mirena IUD may be a good option to control heavy uterine bleeding, although problematic spotting may occur [28].

For adolescents with chronic renal failure without complications, estrogen-containing contraceptives are a good choice, as menstrual flow is regulated, the risk of anemia is lessened, and the process of bone resorption is reversed.

For transplant patients, data about contraceptive method are lacking. In transplant patients who are medically stable, estrogen-containing methods may be used but need to be monitored closely. DMPA or barrier contraception is also an option. The Mirena IUD should not be the first choice for transplant recipients on immunosuppressive agents, as it may carry a higher risk of sexually transmitted infection (STI) than other available forms of contraception.

Pulmonary

As a result of aggressive early and persistent medical care, patients with cystic Fibrosis (CF) are living longer into adulthood. A higher infertility rate exists for women with CF, but sexually active girls still have the potential for pregnancy with its known health risks. Hormonal contraception appears to be a safe alternative for the teenager with CF. Potentially, the progestin component in OCPs, OrthoEvra, and DMPA may thicken bronchial mucus as it does cervical mucus, but this is not a contraindication for using these hormonal methods. The clinician needs to be aware of the rare occurrence of a pulmonary embolus in girls on combination estrogen/progestin contraception. A pulmonary exacerbation in CF patients needs to be differentiated from this medical condition. CF in itself is not a contraindication for the Mirena IUD, but no specific indications are known. Barrier contraception is another option for this group of teenagers.

Gastrointestinal illness

Teenagers with Crohn's disease or ulcerative colitis (inflammatory bowel disease [IBD) may be amenorrheic from nutritional deficits or chronic stress; however, as their status improves, they often resume menstruation. Pregnancy is known potentially to worsen the gastrointestinal symptoms of IBD. Many teenagers with IBD report worsening of the colitis symptoms around the time of menses, perhaps as a result of higher prostaglandins levels causing uterine and colonic musculature contractions. Hormonal contraception can reduce the flare-up of perimenstrual colitis symptoms and anemia associated with IBD. OrthoEvra may be a superior choice in hormonal contraception over OCPs in adolescents with IBD by allowing the teenager to avoid an additional daily oral medication. In addition, if there is active colitis, absorption of the OCP may be reduced, resulting in lowered effectiveness and breakthrough bleeding. DMPA can induce anovulation and amenorrhea, which can eliminate symptoms of dysmenorrhea and anemia. Bone mass issues need to be considered if choosing DMPA [29].

A small number of those with Crohn's disease and ulcerative colitis have coagulation disorders making DMPA a more prudent hormonal option. In all adolescents with IBD, barrier methods are safe. The Mirena IUD may prove to be an excellent option for girls with IBD and hypercoagulability, but as yet, it has not been evaluated in this group.

Teenagers with active liver disease or cirrhosis should not take estrogen-containing medication. The hormonal steroids estrogen and nor-progestins are metabolized in the liver and alter hepatocellular function. Changes include elevation of cholesterol level, reduction in bile acid, changes in bile composition, and reduced volume of biliary secretion [30]. If hepatocellular enzymes return to normal values, OCPs or OrthoEvra may be initiated safely. DMPA may be considered if bleeding is not a concern. The Mirena IUD and barrier methods are other options for adolescents with active or quiescent liver disease.

Hematologic and oncologic problems

Sickle cell anemia is an autosomal recessive genetic disorder, occurring primarily in the United States in African Americans, in which there is a structural red blood cell deformity. Pain crisis occurs when, in the presence of low oxygen levels, the abnormal red cells sickle, then cluster, leading to vaso-occlusion of tissue and potential ischemia. This is not a thrombotic process, and, theoretically, OCPs should not influence the incidence of vaso-occlusive crises. Studies comparing thromboembolic risk in women with and without sickle cell anemia on OCPs have not been done. Contraceptive choice needs to be weighed against the increased maternal and fetal risk of pregnancy in adolescents with sickle cell disease. DMPA has been shown to lessen the incidence of pain crises in women with sickle cell anemia and would be an excellent choice for those patients who need contraception [31]. Barrier methods are another option for adolescents with sickle cell anemia.

Thromboembolic or hypercoagulable states are uncommon in adolescents but merit careful consideration when deciding upon a contraceptive method. Etiologies for thromboses include deficiencies in protein S, protein C, and antithrombin III, or factor V Leiden mutation. A positive family history of a thrombotic event in a relative under age 50 years or a history of venous thromboembolism in the adolescent herself mandates a detailed hematologic investigation. This hematologic evaluation should not be done routinely on all girls starting estrogen/progestin combination contraception, unless other predisposing factors exist. Those with a history of venous thrombosis are at high risk for a subsequent embolic event, so they should not take OCPs or OrthoEvra unless they are anticoagulated. DMPA contains only progestin and does not biochemically affect the clotting factors. A history of a deep vein thrombosis, however, is listed in DMPA packaging as a contraindication to its use. The American College of Obstetrics and Gynecology supports the use of DMPA in women with prior venous thrombosis [32]. More investigations of the newer OCPs, Ortho-Evra, and DMPA may help clarify safety practice guidelines. The Mirena IUD may be an excellent option for teenagers with thrombosis or hypercoagulability, but it has not been evaluated for this group. For now, a safe and effective choice for pregnancy prevention in an adolescent with a tendency for thrombosis is barrier contraception.

Autoimmune disease

Systemic lupus erythematosus (SLE) is a multi-system autoimmune disorder. Menstruating girls with SLE are fertile, and pregnancy is high risk with potential maternal and fetal morbidity. Teenagers with SLE complicated by vasculitis, nephritis, or antiphospholipid antibodies should not take estrogen because of the increased risk of thrombosis. Progestin-only contraception such as DMPA is safe and does not increase this risk. In an adolescent with SLE who has stable disease and no active vasculitis, DMPA is the best choice for contraception, but, in selected patients, OCPs may be used with caution [33]. Barrier methods are safe options for girls with SLE.

Rheumatoid arthritis may result in significant joint immobility and impaired dexterity. Barrier methods may be too physically challenging for the teenager with disabling arthritis. Hormonal methods likely would be the contraception of choice for these adolescents. These include OCPs, OrthoEvra, DMPA, and possibly the Mirena IUD.

Immobility

An adolescent may have a chronic illness that leads to a very sedentary or wheelchair-dependent life. In addition, teenagers may have orthopedic, neurologic, medical, or surgical conditions that render them non-ambulatory. Use of estrogen-containing contraception is contraindicated in these adolescents because of the increased risk of venous thromboembolism. A prospective study found that postoperative women on low-dose OCPs had twice the risk of venous thromboembolism compared with non-OCP users. Furthermore, the estrogen effects on coagulation took up to 6 weeks to resolve after stopping the OCP. Therefore, in preparation for a surgical procedure, OCPs should be discontinued for two cycles before the nonambulatory postoperative period. A progesterone-only method could be instituted at the time the OCPs are stopped to provide adequate contraception for these girls. Because barrier methods may be too physically difficult to be self-inserted or used effectively, DMPA would be one contraceptive choice for those adolescents who are nonambulatory. A significant concern for long-term use of DMPA in these immobile patients is that of lowered bone density. The Mirena IUD may provide the solution for this problem; however, the insertion process may be more challenging depending on the patient's particular anatomical limitations. This has not been studied for this group of patients, but would, in theory, be an effective, safe contraceptive method.

Mental retardation

Mental retardation is associated with delayed psychosexual development; however, over time, these adolescents are fertile and can experience sexual desires and feelings. Pregnancy prevention must be addressed with the teenager and the caretaker, and choice of method should be individualized. Barrier methods are often not appropriate, as they require both manual dexterity and a certain level of cognitive functioning to use these effectively. OCPs and the OrthoEvra patch are contraceptive options if the adolescent is of adequate intelligence or supervised by a responsible adult. Interactions between estrogen/progestin and other prescription medications should be evaluated for the adolescent. DMPA is a popular method for mentally retarded adolescents. The initial adverse effect of vaginal spotting often resolves after an atrophic endometrium is attained, leading to amenorrhea. Amenorrhea from DMPA is a favorable effect for some caretakers, as hygiene issues for a menstruating adolescent who has developmental delay is often a challenge. Weight gain from DMPA can sometimes be limited by implementing nutritional preventive measures. The new black-box warning by the FDA emphasizing the risk of osteopenia may limit long-term use in this population. Sterilization is an option for some adolescents with mental retardation. State laws vary on this issue. A teenager should have exhausted all available medical options for contraception before considering surgical sterilization.

Other medications

As noted in previous sections, anticonvulsants and some psychiatric medications can alter the hepatic metabolism of the estrogen/progestin component of OCPs, rendering them less effective as contraception [20]. A clinician needs to consider these complex dynamics, and prescribe either a different contraceptive agent (such as DMPA), use an OCP with 50 µg of EE, or prescribe a secondary barrier method in case of failure of the hormonal medication. Data for actual effectiveness of higher-dose OCPs for pregnancy prevention are lacking.

Girls taking concurrent antibiotics have a potential for reduced effectiveness of OCPs. In various pharmacologic studies, women on OCPs taking tetracycline, doxycycline, ampicillin, metronidazole, and quinolones do not have lower serum estrogen or progesterone levels. Women prescribed rifampin or griseofulvin, however, have lower serum estrogen and progesterone concentrations on OCPs and are at higher risk of pregnancy from contraception failure. Adolescents on rifampin or griseofulvin should be prescribed DMPA or use barrier methods for contraception [20].

Summary

Adolescents with chronic illness are surviving into adulthood, and the contraceptive needs of this diverse group of girls should be addressed. Teens with chronic illness and medical disabilities progress through the stages of adolescent psychosocial and pubertal development, although the latter may be delayed slightly. These girls interact with peers in a social manner, and they may not receive the contraceptive counseling they require. It can be challenging to find the appropriate contraception for a medically ill teenager; however, pregnancy in many of these girls carries with it the risk of significant morbidity and mortality.

Adolescents with chronic medical illness may be disabled, but they should be allowed to be active participants in their social development and sexual behavior. The clinician needs to be knowledgeable about which contraception is safe and effective for particular illnesses, and needs to have open dialog with all adolescents about pregnancy and prevention of STIs. The contraceptive options available should be individualized for each girl. An adolescent with a chronic illness on a selected contraceptive should be monitored diligently to identify any adverse effects. Many contraceptive choices are available for teens with chronic illness, and more likely will be available in the future.

References

[1] Heroux K. Contraceptive choices in medically ill adolescents. Semin Reprod Med 2003; 21(4):389–98.

[2] Suris JC, Resnick MD, Cassuto N, Blum RW. Sexual behavior of adolescents with chronic disease and disability. J Adolesc Health 1996;19(2):124–31.

[3] Mattson RH, Rebar RW. Contraceptive methods for women with neurologic disorders. Am J Obstet Gynecol 1993;168:2027–32.

[4] Collaborative Group for the Study of Stroke in Young Women. Associated risk factors. JAMA 1975;231:718–22.

[5] Heroux K. Contraceptive choices in medically ill adolescents. Semin Reprod Med 2003; 21(4):389–98.

[6] Neinstein L, Katz B. Contraceptive use in the chronically ill adolescent female. Part II. J Adolesc Health Care 1986;7(5):350–60.

[7] Crawford P. Interactions between antiepileptic drugs and hormonal contraception. CNS Drugs 2002;16:263–72.

[8] Back DJ, Orne ML. Pharmacokinetic drug interactions with oral contraceptives. Clin Pharmacokinet 1990;18:472–84.

[9] Crawford P, Chadwick DJ, Martin C, et al. The interaction of ohenytoin and carbamazepine with combined oral contraceptive steroids. Br J Clin Pharmacol 1990;30:892–6.

[10] Saano V, et al. Effects of felbamate on the pharmacokinetics of a low-dose combination oral contraceptive. Clin Pharmacol Ther 1995;58:523–31.

[11] Rosenfeld WE, et al. Effect of topiramate on the pharmacokinetics of an oral contraceptive containing norethindrone and ethinyl estradiol in patients with epilepsy. Epilepsia 1997; 38:317–23.

[12] Crawford P, et al. The lack of effect of sodium valproate on the pharmacokinetics of oral contraceptive steroids. Contraception 1986;33:23–9.

[13] Eldon MA, et al. Gabapentin does not interact with a contraceptive regimen of norethindrone acetate and ethinyl estradiol. Neurology 1998;50:1146–8.

[14] Mengel HB, Houston A, Back DJ. An evaluation of the interaction between tiagabine and oral contraceptives in female volunteers. Journal of Pharmaceutical Medicine 1994;4:141–50.

[15] Natsch S, Hekster YA, Keyser A, et al. Newer anticonvulsant drugs: role of Pharmacology, drug interactions and adverse reactions in drug choice. Drug Saf 1997;17:228–40.

[16] Holmes LB, Harvey EA, Coull BA, et al. The teratogenicity of anticonvulsant drugs. N Engl J Med 2001;344:1132–8.

[17] Sapire EK. Depo Provera and carbamazepine [letter]. Br J Fam Plann 1990;15:130.

[18] Mattson R, Rebar R. Contraceptive method for women with neurological disorders. Am J Obstet Gynecol 1993;168:2027–32.

[19] Kaunitz AM, Mestman J. Hormonal contraception in women with common medical conditions: Benefits and risk of use. Dialogues Contracept 2004;8(6):1–7.

[20] American College of Obstetricians and Gynecologists. The use of hormonal contraception in women with coexisting medical conditions. ACOG Practice Bulletin 2000;18:1–13.

[21] Spellacy WN, Tsibris JC, Hunter-Bonner DL, et al. Six-month carbohydrate metabolism studies in women using oral contraceptives containing gestodene and ethinyl estradiol. Contraception 1992;45(6):533–9.

[22] Frederiksen M. Depot medroxy progesterone acetate concentration in women with medical problems. J Reprod Med 1996;41:414–8.

[23] Heroux K. Contraceptive choices in medically ill adolescents. Semin Reprod Med 2003; 21(4):389–98.

[24] Cardoso F, Polonia J, Santos A, et al. Low-dose oral contraceptives and 24-hour ambulatory blood pressure. Int J Gynaecol Obstet 1997;59:237–43.

[25] WHO Collaborative Study of Cardiovascular Disease and Steroid Hormone Contraception. Ischemic stroke and combined oral contraceptives: results of an international, multi-centre, case-control study. Lancet 1996;348:498–505.

[26] Sidney S, Siscovick DS, Petitti DB, et al. Myocardial infarction and use of low-dose oral contraceptives: a pooled analysis of 2 US studies. Circulation 1998;98:1058–63.

[27] Schwartz SM, Petitti DB, Siscovick DS, et al. Stroke and the use of low-dose oral contraceptives in young women: a pooled analysis of two US studies. Stroke 1998;29:2277–84.

[28] Andersson JK, Rybo G. Levonorgestrel-releasing intrauterine device in the treatment of menorrhagia. Br J Obstet Gynaecol 1990;97:690–4.

[29] Cromer BA, Blair JM, Mahan JD, et al. A prospective comparison of bone density in adolescent girls receiving depot medroxyprogesterone acetate (Depo Provera), levonorgestrel (Norplant), and oral contraceptives. J Pediatr 1996;129:671–6.

[30] Khoo SK, Correy JF. Contraception and the high risk woman. Med J Aust 1981;1:60–8.

[31] Robinson GE, Burren T, Mackie IJ, et al. Changes in haemostasis after stopping the combined contraceptive pill: Implications for major surgery. BMJ 1991;302:269–71.

[32] Frederiksen M. Depot medroxy progesterone acetate concentration in women with medical problems. J Reprod Med 1996;41:414–8.

[33] Petri M, Robinson C. Oral contraceptives and systemic lupus erythematosis. Arthritis Rheum 1997;40:797–803.

ELSEVIER
SAUNDERS

Adolesc Med 16 (2005) 645–663

ADOLESCENT
MEDICINE
CLINICS

Contraceptive Issues of Youth and Adolescents in Developing Countries: Highlights from the Philippines and Other Asian Countries

Emma Alesna-Llanto, MD, FPPS[a],*,
Corazon M. Raymundo, MA, MS, DSc[b]

[a]*Department of Pediatrics, College of Medicine-Philippine General Hospital,
University of the Philippines Manila, Taft Avenue, Manila, Philippines 1000*
[b]*Population Institute, University of the Philippines, Diliman, Quezon City, Philippines*

In 2000, there were about 1.15 billion adolescents, comprising about 20% of the world's population. The proportion of adolescents in the population varies little from region to region in the developing world, from about 19% in Asia to 23% in Africa. By 2020, there will be 65 million more adolescents, with Africa and Asia projected to contribute most to this rapidly growing segment of the population [1].

Eighty-seven percent of adolescents live in developing countries where poverty is deep and pervasive. Almost 25% (238 million) subsist on less than $1 a day, and most face the prospects of inadequate education, continued gender inequality, early marriage and childbearing, and the threat of HIV [2]. Diverse factors contribute to this worrying situation. These include a declining age at menarche, an older age at marriage, improved levels of literacy, and a change in cultural values brought about by the effects of globalization, urbanization, and widespread use of communication technologies, high migration rates, and a decline in the prevalence of the extended family. In the 1990s, 294 million adolescents lived in urban centers; in 2025, it is estimated that the number will double to 634 million [3].

* Corresponding author.
E-mail address: teendoc99@yahoo.com (E. Alesna-Llanto).

All these changes impact on the sexual mores and behavior of adolescents. These factors tend to prolong the period between sexual maturation and marriage, providing more opportunities for premarital sex. Traditional customs that discouraged sex before marriage are breaking down. Thus, a substantial number of young people in many countries engage in largely unprotected premarital sex [4].

In most developed countries, most women have sex before age 20 (67% in France, 79% in Great Britain, and 71% in the United States). There is evidence that sexual activity is also common in the developing world. For females, premarital sexual activity varies widely across regions, but some patterns are observable. For instance, rates of sexual activity are concentrated in the 2% to 11% range in various settings in Asia, 12% to 44% in various settings in Latin America by age 16, and 45% to 52% in settings in sub-Saharan Africa by age 19 [5].

As a result, the risk of unwanted pregnancy, abortion, and sexually transmitted disease (STD), including HIV, has increased significantly for adolescents and youth. The consequences of adolescent sexual activity can be gleaned from the statistics gathered by the United Nations Population Fund in 2000 [2]:

- Despite the shift toward later marriage in many parts of the world, 82 million girls in developing countries will marry early [2]. As many as 73% of girls in Bangladesh and 50% in India will marry before they turn 18 [6].
- Fourteen million girls aged 15 to 19—both married and unmarried—give birth each year [2]. In Asia, childbearing occurs soon after marriage and in Bangladesh, 63% of currently married females have given birth; 48% of currently married females in India, and 43% of currently married females in Nepal have given birth [7].
- Worldwide, mostly as a result of unintended pregnancy, nearly 4.5 million adolescents undergo abortion each year; 40% occur under unsafe conditions [2]. In Latin America, and regions in Africa and Asia where abortion is illegal, the overall abortion rate is estimated at 30 per 1000 pregnancies, higher than in Australia and the United States (22 to 23 per 1000 pregnancies), where abortion is legal [8].
- Pregnancy is a leading cause of death for women aged 15 to 19 years, and this is because of complications of childbirth and unsafe abortion. Girls aged 15 to 19 are twice as likely to die in childbirth as are those in their 20s; girls under 15 are five times as likely as those in their 20s [2]. Only 25% of all women in Bangladesh, Nepal, and Pakistan receive prenatal care; less than 10% of women in Bangladesh and Nepal deliver with the help of a trained attendant. The scenario is worsened by the high incidence of anemia. In developing countries, the chances of dying from the complications of pregnancy, childbirth, and abortion are 1 in 65; in developed countries, the chances are 1 in 2125 [9].
- For every woman who dies, between 30 and 100 more live with a painful disability; it was estimated that about 2 million women live with obstetric fistulas [10].

• The World Health Organization (WHO) estimates that at least one third of more than 333 million new cases of curable sexually transmitted infections (STIs) each year occur among people under age 25. Young adults aged 15 to 24 years account for 50% of the approximately 5 million new cases of HIV infection each year. At the end of 2001, an estimated 11.8 million young people were living with HIV; 62% were female, and 38% were males. Only 2% of affected youth lived in industrialized countries; 72% alone were from the sub-Saharan countries [11].

Adolescents need to protect themselves from unintended pregnancies and infection. Although abstaining from sexual relations remains a primary means of prevention, sexually active adolescents need effective contraceptives to avert pregnancies and unsafe abortion. According to the WHO, young age does not constitute a medical reason to avoid any contraceptive method [12]. There is no evidence that provision of information about contraception results in increased rates of sexual activity, earlier age at first intercourse, or more partners. Conversely, there is no evidence that refusal to provide contraception results in abstinence or postponement of sexual relations [13].

Undoubtedly, the sexual and contraceptive behavior of this cohort of adolescents will have an impact not only on their own health and well-being but also on the future population growth and economic development of their respective countries and regions. It also is apparent that discussions about contraception need to stress the importance of protection from pregnancy and STIs, including HIV.

Most young people in developing counties who are in urgent need of contraceptive services, however, face formidable obstacles in accessing these services. To formulate programs that will be responsive to their unique needs, it is critical to gain insight into adolescents' knowledge, misconceptions, use, and the dynamics that govern use, barriers that they face, and their unmet needs. This article highlights contraceptive issues in Asia, home to some 700 million adolescents [1]. The region is composed of Bangladesh, India, Nepal, Pakistan and Sri-Lanka in South Asia and Indonesia, Thailand and the Philippines in Southeast Asia. South Asia has 106 million young people living in extreme poverty, the largest concentration in the world [2]. The article starts with a description of the socio–cultural milieu of Asian adolescents, their knowledge and use of contraceptives, barriers to contraceptive use, and a description of current efforts to broaden contraceptive availability.

Vignettes and experiences of youth of the Philippines will be used to highlight certain reproductive and contraceptive issues. The Philippines, like most developing countries, is experiencing a youth bulge, with 15 million adolescents making up 22% of its population [14]. Filipino adolescents are growing up in a society buffeted by opposing forces: Westernization and urbanization on one hand and conservative religious and traditional values on the other. Data on the Philippines were obtained from the findings of the Young Adults Fertility Survey, YAFS 2 (1994) and YAFS 3 (2002).

Understanding the socio–cultural and economic milieu of adolescents in the developing world

In developing countries where resources are scarce, difficulties in contraceptive access go beyond logistics. Social norms that dictate the role of men and women have a direct influence on sexual behavior, contraceptive use, and the balance of responsibility for childbearing. To be able to understand the contraceptive behaviors of adolescents, it is necessary to understand their social milieu.

Gender inequality

In Asian societies, boys are favored over girls. Thus, parents tend to invest less on the health, nutritional, and educational needs of girls. Although 80% of girls are enrolled in secondary school in Thailand, Sri Lanka, and the Philippines, 70% to 76% of girls in Bangladesh, Pakistan, and Nepal remain illiterate [15].

Several factors are responsible for girls' lower level of secondary school enrollment: parents' perception that education is more beneficial for their sons, limited job options for women in sectors demanding higher education, and worries about girls' safety outside the village [3]. Lack of educational opportunities for girls, poverty, dowry, and the sense that the main value of girls is as wives and mothers, are factors that lead to early marriage [6].

In comparison to women, the mean age of marriage of Asian men is between 23 and 25 years [16]. The age gap has far-reaching implications. Young girls who marry older, more sexually experienced men expose themselves to the perils of early childbearing and STI/ HIV. Young brides often share no power in the relationship; thus they are generally unable to negotiate condom use or to refuse sexual relations. With curtailment of decision making, mobility, education, and job opportunities, young married women often do not seek health care without the permission of their husbands nor can they afford to pay for services on their own [17].

Gender roles

On the whole, Asian societies fervently adhere to the age-old double standards; premarital sexual activity is more prevalent among Asian males. From case studies gathered by Brown, gender disparities were widest in Asia, where reported rates were at least five times as high among males compared with females. In the Latin American case studies, rates were up to twice as high among males as among females [18]. The societies that tolerate premarital sex among males bestow tremendous cultural value on virginity for women. Females also generally are expected to be submissive, and thus the decision to use contraception is viewed as the male's prerogative [19].

Cases studies offer a glimpse on how traditional gender roles limit the decision making of women regarding consent, timing of sexual intercourse, and negotiation for contraception. A study among rural adolescents in Thailand showed that for males, leading motives for first sex were curiosity, physical need, and peer pressure. Among females, the leading reasons were love and the desire to strengthen a committed relationship. Girls also expressed fears of losing their partner, provoking his anger, or endangering the relationship as important factors that prevented them from exercising choice in the timing of sexual activity [18]. Among Filipino girls, the first partner was a boyfriend 85% of the time, while among males, 46% had sex with a casual acquaintance, and 7.7% had their sexual debut with a commercial sex worker. About 48.9% of males eventually had multiple sex partners. Not all sexual debuts were wanted. At least 6% of girls and 1% of boys said that they were forced to have sex [20].

Negotiation for contraception is untenable in the context of nonconsensual or forced sex. Data on sexual coercion among youth in developing countries are limited. At the global consultative meeting on Nonconsensual Sexual Experiences of Young People in Developing Countries in New Delhi in September of 2003, however, studies showed that 15% to 30% of sexually active girls reported coercion during sexual debut; fewer than 10% of boys reported forced first sex [21].

Poverty and reproductive health

Poverty casts a long, ugly shadow on the reproductive health of young people. In most countries, young women from the poorest households were more likely than those from the richest households to enter into early marriage and childbearing and least likely to use maternal health services, to know how to prevent sexual transmission of HIV, and to be practicing contraception. They were often illiterate and lived in rural areas with little access to reproductive health programs [22].

Poverty also breeds transactional sex, in which an adolescent is powerless to use contraception. Impoverished adolescent girls hook up with sugar daddies who offer money for school fees, meals, and gifts in exchange for sex. Once in these relationships with older men, girls have little power to negotiate the use of condoms [11,23]. The situation is even more desperate for prostituted youth and street children as young as 7 or 8 year olds engaged in survival sex [24].

In countries where unemployment is high, young women migrate to urban centers or go abroad to seek low-paying jobs that expose them to sexual exploitation. In 2001, there were more than 6000 Filipino overseas workers in the teenage group, four out five being females. They were recruited as domestic workers, factory workers, or nightclub dancers in Japan and other Asian countries [24].

Contraceptive knowledge and use among adolescents in the developing world

Knowledge about contraceptive methods among married adolescents

Over 90% of married Asian adolescents have heard of at least one traditional or modern method of contraception. Knowledge was highest in Bangladesh, at

99.7%. Although more than 90% of teenage women in most countries in Asia, North Africa, the Near East, Latin America, and the Caribbean were aware of at least one contraceptive method, in sub-Saharan Africa, knowledge was generally low [4].

Adolescents' knowledge of a specific method was related to the method mix endorsed in their country. In India, for instance, the most commonly recognized was tubal ligation (89%), which is the predominant method being promoted. In Vietnam, the most well known modern method among urban youth was the intrauterine device (IUD) [7].

Condom knowledge, attitudes and misconceptions

Knowledge of condoms among adolescents is of particular interest, because it is the one method that provides dual protection from pregnancy and STDs. Among married female adolescents in Asia, condom knowledge had a wide variation, from 18% in Pakistan, 48% in Sri-Lanka, to 53% in Indonesia. Condom knowledge was highest in Thailand (89%) and the Philippines (85%) [7]. Specific information about the condom's benefits are lacking, however, as illustrated by the findings among Filipino males:

> Although 97.6% of sexually active Filipino male respondents know of condom, not all were aware of the benefits of proper and consistent condom use. Thirty-six percent did not know that condoms can prevent HIV/AIDS; 26% did not know that condoms can protect against STD, while 16% did not know that condoms can prevent pregnancy [25].

Among those who know the benefits, many misconceptions prevail. In a study of secondary school students in Nairobi and Kenya, most young people were aware of the condom's role in HIV prevention but were mistrustful of its efficacy. Among the misconceptions: the HIV virus is small to pass through the pores; condoms burst during use or remain in the vagina or climb into the womb [18]. Besides the misinformation, young males held negative attitudes that could shape behavior. Among Filipino males, the use of condoms also has cultural and gender-specific connotations:

> Condoms are often connected with HIV/AIDS infection and prevention, not contraception. Condoms are traditionally associated with illicit sex; thus condoms are dirty and shouldn't be used with girlfriends or wives [26]. Filipino youth believe that condoms make sexual intercourse less pleasurable (58%); respondent would be too embarrassed to buy condom at store (47%); condoms are too expensive for regular use (34%), and use of condoms is against religion (32%) [25].

Contraceptive use among married female adolescents

Contraceptive use varies markedly by region and country. Only 13% of married adolescents ages 15 to 19 use contraception in sub-Saharan Africa, compared with 55% in Latin America and the Caribbean. In Latin America and the Caribbean, 11% of married adolescents in Haiti use contraception, compared with 51% in Colombia. Wide variations also are seen in Asia. It varies from 6.2% in Pakistan to 44.5% in Indonesia [3]. Modern methods usually used by youth include condoms, oral contraceptive pills (OCPs), and hormonal injections. Traditional methods include the calendar or rhythm method, herbal methods, and withdrawal.

In general, married adolescents used modern contraceptive methods more often than traditional methods. The use of modern methods was as high as 44% in Indonesia and as low as 2.4% in Pakistan (Table 1). The most commonly used by married adolescents mirrored the method promoted in their country. Until recently, the national planning programs of India and Vietnam promoted female sterilization and IUDs, respectively. It should be noted that condom use is low, with only 1% to 2% of married adolescents using the method.

The 2003 United Nations Population Fund (UNFPA) global survey indicated that emergency contraception is now available in 65 countries, including India, Nepal, and Pakistan. More than 19 million female condoms have been supplied in more than 70 countries worldwide. A study that included Indonesia found that the female condom is most acceptable where the female condom is considered preferable to the male version and where men already accept contraception and believe that their peers support the method [27]. No studies on emergency contraception, the female condom, injectable contraceptives, and implants among Asian adolescents were accessed, however. In the Philippines, there are also doubts that implants that involve minor surgery will have many takers, because the procedure is not culturally acceptable [26].

Although rates are low in Asia, there are indications that more adolescent women are starting to use modern contraception. Basing on data from the 1970s, rates have doubled or tripled in Indonesia, the Philippines, and Thailand. The increase in Bangladesh has been 10-fold, from a 2% to 20% [6].

Table 1

Percentage of married female adolescents using contraceptives in countries in South Asia and Southeast Asia, according to type of method and most preferred modern method

| Country | Percentage of adolescents using | | | Most preferred modern method |
	Any method	Traditional method	Modern method	
Bangladesh (1997)	32.9	4.9	27.8	Pill, 18%
India (1998–1999)	8.0	3.3	4.7	BTL, 2%
Nepal (1996)	6.5	2.2	4.4	Condom 2.2%
Pakistan (1996–1997)	6.2	3.9	2.4	Condom, 1%
Sri-Lanka (1987)	20.2	9.5	10.7	Pill, 7%
Indonesia (1997)	44.5	0.2	44.3	Injectable, 24%
Philippines (1998)	21.8	10.4	11.4	Pill, 6%
Thailand (1987)	43.0	2.6	40.5	Pill 25%
Vietnam (1997)	18.1	3.2	14.9	IUD, 10%

Data from Pachauri S, Santhya KG. Reproductive choices for Asian adolescents: a focus on contraceptive behavior. Int Fam Plann Perspect 2002;28(4):186–95; with permission.

Contraception use rates among married adolescents compared with their 20- to 24-year-old counterparts are definitely lower. There was a 10 to 20 percentage point difference between the two age groups; the difference is most pronounced in Vietnam and least in Pakistan. This pattern denoted not only a lower level of sexual activity among adolescents but also the fact that many are just beginning child-bearing and are less inclined to delay or avoid pregnancy than older women [7].

Discontinuation and contraceptive switching

There is little information on whether adolescents switch to another method immediately after discontinuing a contraceptive. Such information is needed to design appropriate services for adolescents who need special information, counseling, and follow-up care. Discontinuing contraceptives leaves adolescents vulnerable to unwanted pregnancies and unsafe abortion.

There are few data on discontinuation, but in countries with relatively high contraceptive prevalence, such as Indonesia and Bangladesh, adolescents tended to discontinue their method within the first year of use compared with older women, They were also two to three times more inclined to give up contraceptive use because of adverse effects, health concerns, desire for more effective and convenient method, problems with access, or their husband's disapproval. Adolescents, however, were no more likely to discontinue use because of method failure. In India, compared with women aged 25 or older, adolescents were more likely to cite desire for a child rather than mention method failure as their main reason for abandoning contraception [7].

Data on contraceptive switching are just as scarce. A pregnancy scare often prompts adolescents to either initiate use or to switch to a more reliable method. This may prove difficult, however, because of a general reluctance to approach a health facility and unfamiliarity with the system. Among adult women in the Philippines, the reasons for switching were: inappropriate medical service, unavailability of some methods and supplies, and inconvenience. Women from Indonesia and Turkey often mentioned adverse effects as the top reason for switching to other methods. It was noted that switching was more common among women who were better educated, urbanized, and had higher contraceptive awareness [28]. Contraceptive switching is also higher among highly educated and younger women in the United States. Their reasons for switching, however, were not related to supplies or services, but rather with level and duration of contraceptive effectiveness, health risks, and STD prevention [29]. Because adolescents tend to discontinue a method because of exaggerated fears of adverse effects, they should be given accurate information about expected adverse effects and offered alternatives should they decide to switch methods [30].

Contraception among unmarried adolescents

There are scant data on use of contraception among unmarried Asian adolescents, because most surveys limit questions about contraceptive use to currently married women only. Data are available for few countries: the Philippines, Kazakhstan, Kyrgystan, Uzbekistan, and Papua New Guinea. The proportions of unmarried women reporting contraceptive use in these five countries varies from 1% to 2% in the Philippines and Uzbekistan to 12% in Kazakhstan [31]. A review of studies from India, Vietnam, and the Philippines indicate that most unmarried, sexually active adolescents do not use a contraceptive method. Those who do use a method often report use of traditional methods that are unreliable and likely to be difficult for adolescents [7]. The calendar method for instance, needs accurate knowledge of the reproductive cycle and active cooperation of the partner.

Among unmarried Filipino adolescents, only 21% used any kind of contraception. Among those who did, only 50% used a reliable method (condom and OCP), while almost 40% practiced withdrawal. Among males, 41.3% used a condom, and among females, 15.1% used OCPs. In general, the level of practice of contraception during the last sexual intercourse increased, and the difference is accounted for by OCPs (15.1% to 28.5); on the other hand, condom use by males declined (39.8% to 32.7%). Increased use of OCPs implies that women became more proactive in pregnancy prevention after sexual debut. Contraceptive use was low, even with a commercial sex worker, with only 50% of respondents reporting condom use [20].

Reasons cited for nonuse include: did not expect to have sex (49%), did not think pregnancy was possible with one intercourse (34%), did not know about contraception (15%). Other reasons included: partner objection and concerns that contraceptives are dangerous to health and remove fun from sex [25].

Barriers to contraception

In a study among 653 young Filipino women who had induced abortions, the following reasons were cited for nonuse of contraceptives: fear of adverse effects/ health reasons (47.6%), never heard/did not know where to source (20.8), did not feel it was needed (8.4%), husband/ relatives objected (4.7%), religious reasons (0.9%). [32]

Among youth who used condoms, the mean travel time from respondents' home to condom source was 27 minutes for an urban youth and 58 minutes for an adolescent in rural areas. The most common source was a pharmacy or store, unlike adults who obtained contraceptive supplies from the public sector (government hospitals or health centers). This may be explained by the fact that youth are not the target clientele of the family planning program [25].

Adolescents, both married and unmarried, face numerous barriers to contraceptive access. Among the barriers are:

societal and familial pressure to have a child soon after marriage

- Gender inequality
- Social stigma

- Religions that do not approve of modern methods
- Lack of information about contraception and reproductive health in general
- Misconceptions about side effects
- Social stigma and judgmental attitudes of health providers
- Lack of youth friendly services
- Inappropriate services

The situation in the Philippines illustrates potential barriers to providing contraceptive services among the young. Although the Adolescent and Youth Development Plan has been in place since 2002, implementation of the program has been hindered by lack of funds. The political commitment needed to actualize a reproductive health program for adolescents is apparently absent. This can be discerned from the administration's adamant support only for natural methods. Without the crucial support from the president and the Department of Health, the promotion of modern methods has been lacking, left largely to the discretion of local government officials. Another urgent problem is that of dwindling contraceptive supplies. United States Agency for International Development (USAID) and UNFPA, which supply 80% of the Philippines' contraceptives. will withdraw their support by 2007. The greatest impact will be on the poor, who are totally dependent on free contraceptive supplies [33].

Lack of other supportive legislative measures also makes providing contraceptive services to adolescents difficult. Philippine Medical jurisprudence does not include confidentiality or informed consent among adolescent patients, an element essential in the delivery of adolescent health services [34,35]. Philippine Law does not recognize the concept of mature minor [36]. In contrast, in developed countries like the United States, adolescents can obtain contraception and treatment for STDs without parental consent [37].

The Catholic Church in the Philippines is highly politicized and exerts considerable pressure against legislation (and their proponents) that promotes modern methods. Such was the fate of the Reproductive Health Care Act of 2002 that called for the creation of "comprehensive, age-specific" health programs. It was the subject of an intense and emotional lobby by pro-life groups that claimed that it promoted promiscuity and abortion. Wary congressmen rejected the original version and continue to sit on the modified bill [38].

There is a pervasive fear that providing sexuality education automatically leads promiscuity among young people. Filipino adolescents said that parents are appropriate sources of information, but most parents are not well informed or equipped with the proper the communication skills to be effective [39]. School does little to fill the knowledge gap. It is not surprising then that media and peers have become main sources of information on sexuality, hardly the best sources for accurate, gender-sensitive information [40]. As a result, youth are ignorant and misinformed about critical issues. For instance, 25% think HIV is curable, and 60% think that there is no chance that they will ever get infected. [25]

Table 2
Percentage of currently married female adolescents with unmet need for contraception in selected countries in south Asia and Southeast Asia

Country and survey year	Unmet need			Percentage of demand satisfied
	Spacing	Limiting	Total	
Bangladesh (1997)	17.8	0.9	18.7	65
India (1998–99)	25.6	1.6	27.1	22.8
Nepal (1996)	38.9	1.6	40.5	13.9
Pakistan (1996–97)	22.4	0.6	23.0	21.4
Indonesia (1997)	8.6	0.5	9.1	83.2
Philippines (1998)	27.4	4.6	32.1	41.4
Vietnam (1997)	9.0	0.7	9.7	65.1

Data from Pachauri S, Santhya KG. Reproductive choices for Asian adolescents: a focus on contraceptive behavior. Int Fam Plann Perspect 2002;28(4):186–95; with permission.

Unmet needs

Overall, 82% of all adolescent pregnancies are unintended [30]. Among married adolescents in Asian countries, the proportion of unplanned births varied from 37% in the Philippines, 30% in Thailand, Sri-Lanka and Nepal, 21% in Bangladesh, to about 10% in Pakistan and Indonesia. Most unplanned births were mistimed rather than unwanted, indicating a significant unmet need for contraception. If sexually active unmarried teens were included in surveys, the statistics for unmet need would be higher [7].

The proportion of unmet needs among married adolescents was highest in Nepal, at 40.5% and lowest in Indonesia, at less than 10%. Most of the unmet need among this population was for a way to space births rather than as a means of limiting childbearing. It can be gleaned from the data that current family planning programs did not adequately answer the contraceptive needs of most adolescents in India, Nepal, Pakistan, and the Philippines (Table 2).

The high unmet need, coupled with a high contraceptive knowledge, is evidence that married adolescents face barriers to contraceptive use. Youth have articulated the need to deal with gaps in reproductive health services. Among predominantly Catholic Filipino youth, 95% believe the government should provide family planning services, and 69% believe that family planning services should be available to adolescents. Moreover, 39% predicted that decision to access these services will not be affected by religion. [20]

Expanding contraceptive options and access

For young people to be able to protect themselves against pregnancy and STIs, they need information, skills, and products. Research has shown that effective sexuality education includes not only information, but also involves making services available and accessible to young people. Programs should teach skills in decision-making and enhance health-seeking behaviors.

A 1998 review of programs in the Asia-Pacific region showed that the focus of most family planning and population programs in the 1970s and 1990s was on married couples of reproductive age. For the youth, programs merely sought to impart information, working on the presumption that knowledge would lead to changes in behavior. Knowledge change was not complemented with appropriate programs and services. Furthermore, programs are ad hoc, small-scale and not interrelated. Programs in most countries have no policy framework, cater to the youth in general, and do not address the needs of various groups. Only few of the countries (Malaysia, Thailand, and the Philippines) did a needs assessment before initiating their interventions. Most of these programs are UNFPA-inspired and funded except for those in Vietnam and Cambodia. The authors concluded with the observation that all of these programs for adolescents and youth were planned and initiated by adults with very little participation from youth, including adolescents [4].

These deficiencies were recognized in the 1990s, resulting in a rethinking of program formulation. The shift in approach was crystallized by the provisions of the International Conference on Population and Development (ICPD), held in 1994 in Cairo, Egypt. The ICPD addressed adolescent reproductive health issues, including unwanted pregnancy, unsafe abortion, and STIs, including HIV, through the promotion of responsible and healthy reproductive and sexual behavior, including voluntary abstinence, and the provision of appropriate services and counseling specifically suited for that age group. It also aimed to substantially reduce all adolescent pregnancies [41].

What needs to be done

Provide access to accurate information

Legal, regulatory, and cultural barriers to sexual and reproductive health information and services for adolescents should be removed. The misconception that that sexuality education will promote promiscuity has hampered efforts to give youth accurate information. To be effective, information/education programs should incorporate several elements [3,7,18,20,32]:

- Programs should target groups with appropriate messages [6].
- Youth not sexually active: abstinence; delay; information about fertility, risks, and future contraceptive use; and self-protection skills
- Sexually active, unmarried youth: secondary abstinence; delay; and information about fertility, risks, and contraceptive services
- Sexually active, married youth: delay first pregnancy, child spacing, and contraceptive services
- Encourage parental involvement and promote adult communication and interaction with adolescents. Case studies indicate that young females and males have different preferences for information sources. Females preferred

information from family (especially mothers), while males preferred the media as their information source [18].

- Behavior change communication (BCC) refers to the various approaches intended to improve knowledge, skills, and attitudes. BCC topics include reproductive biology, human development, relationships and feelings, sexuality, communication and negotiation, gender issues, safer sex practices (including abstinence, delay of first sexual encounter, and limitation of partners), and methods of protection against pregnancy and STIs, including HIV [42].

- Programs that target boys also should be developed. Before the ICPD, programs neglected men's roles, and programs served women almost exclusively. Today, programs such as Mobilizing Young Men to Care in South Africa and the Better Life Options Program for Boys in India seek to change the values behind harmful behaviors [3,42].

- Multiple entry points (school, workplace, sports, and social activities) may be used to broaden the reach of educational programs. Various innovative communication approaches harnessing mass media and the newest communication technology should be used to deliver health information. Some examples of programs initiated in the Philippines serve to illustrate the verve and creativity that are essential in programs for adolescents. As of 2004, The UNFPA -funded Population Commission listed 33 youth programs, such as Dial-A-Friend, Friends Online, Email A Friend, Counseling on Air, Enter Educate Videos, Body Talk TV series, XYZ tri-media campaign, and Kabalaka (folk theater). With a sizeable proportion of youth owning cell phones, text (SMS) messaging has been suggested as a way to reach the youth. Media should be urged to give accurate information and to present adolescents in a more positive light [43].

- Involve parents and community and religious leaders to gain wider acceptance of reproductive health programs. In 1996, the UNFPA with the Department of Health mobilized Muslim religious leaders in Mindanao who provided health information to men, women, and adolescents. After 8 years, the efforts expanded to four more regions in the region, culminating in a historic fatwa or declaration stating Islam's support for reproductive health and family planning [33].

Expand options and access to services and products

Information is only the first step towards preventing unintended pregnancies, abortions, and STDs and HIV. To be effective, educational programs should be linked to services that include contraception, STD and HIV prevention, testing, and pregnancy-related care.

Those who formulate programs should understand that youth is not a homogenous population. The needs of youth from different regions will differ; thus the focus for countries in South Asia where early marriage is the norm is to delay marriage. In Southeast Asia, however, efforts should be directed to limit and space births [7]. Programs should address the social, cultural, and economic obstacles encountered in accessing health service. This is especially true for poor women who marry young, who are illiterate, unemployed, and with limited mobility [22].

Services should be youth-friendly, which means having specially trained health providers, privacy, confidentiality, accessibility, and affordability [3,20,44].

Where resources are scare, programs must build on existing services and provide linkages and referral systems. For example, school-based clinics with no reproductive health facilities may be linked to a clinic in the community that offers these services [3,7,45].

A community-based program is recommended for poor, uneducated young women living in the rural areas who cannot be reached by programs that rely on mass media, clinics, or schools. An alternate delivery strategy such as the use of female outreach workers and community-based distribution of contraceptives to newlyweds may be more suitable [22].

Socially marginalized youth who are extremely vulnerable to sexual exploitation, pregnancy, STI, and HIV also should be provided with services through community-based outreach programs and in the setting of drop-in centers, transitional homes, and shelters [46].

Modern methods available should not be limited to those offered by national family planning programs (eg, sterilization, IUD, and natural family planning), methods that are not appropriate for adolescents. Methods instead should be tailored to the needs of both married and unmarried adolescents [7].

A "basket of services and products" should be offered to allow for a contraceptive mix, because adolescents may shift from one method to another. There also should be an emphasis on the need for dual protection. There should be provisions for emergency contraception, because nonconsensual sex is not uncommon. Counseling should include information on possible adverse effects, because this is one of the most frequent reasons for discontinuing contraceptives [12].

Social marketing can increase access by offering contraceptives at subsidized costs, using innovative, straightforward approaches, and including unmarried adolescents as target clientele [3,4,47]. Social marketing of condoms by DKT International has increased condom use significantly among young men in Vietnam [48]. In the Philippines, "Be hip, be cool, be safe" is the message disseminated through multi-media and nontraditional venues such as concerts, dance, and theater (Kondom Kapers). Frenzy condoms come in different colors and flavors and are sold in pharmacies, supermarkets, neighborhood stores, gasoline stations, motels, bars, and massage parlors [49].

Improve the status of women

Long-term policies and programs must address the underlying social, cultural, and economic factors that contribute to adolescent sexual activity and childbearing. Education has an indelible impact on women's lives. Educated women are more likely to delay marriage and childbearing and have attended deliveries; their babies have better outcomes [13]. All-out efforts should be instituted to eliminate all forms of violence against women and to end human trafficking [3].

Programmatic recommendations

Links should be established between adolescent reproductive health (ARH) programs and other youth activities such as youth development, educational opportunities, job training, and microenterprise [42,47].

Programs should have built-in mechanisms and funding for monitoring and evaluation, including cost-benefit analysis. The long view is to sustain a program and scale up and move beyond localized areas [47]. Different strategies should be explored to assure sustainability

- Cooperation and collaboration between different government and non-government agencies
- Invite the private and commercial sector to contribute ARH programs
- Lobby for long-term donor support
- Coordination between donors and flexible funding mechanisms [20,47]

Swaps, or sector-wide approaches, involves donors coming together to pool funds instead of supporting separate programs [50].

There is little research measuring the impact of reproductive health programs. Efforts are relatively new, and assessment is difficult. Most evidence of successful outcomes in this area was obtained from case studies and reports. Documentation and evaluation of program should be improved [4,42,47].

Youth involvement will engender a sense of ownership. Program design, delivery, and evaluation should include youth in a real, sustained, and meaningful manner [3,4,6,20,47].

Political will, together with coordinated multi-sectoral programs, resulted in the reduction of HIV prevalence in Uganda from its peak at around 15% of adults in 1991 to 5% by 2001 [42]. In Thailand, government determination to enforce the 100% Condom Program in brothels, together with wide access to HIV prevention campaigns and consistent supply of condoms, resulted in lowering HIV infection rates [51].

Investing in the reproductive health of youth in developing countries: what is at stake

The paper Adding It Up summarizes the health and nonhealth benefits of investing in reproductive health in the developing world. The medical benefits of reproductive health services are easy to figure out with statistics, but the contributions to gender equity, economic growth, and poverty alleviation are underestimated by governments and policy makers [52].

Sexual and reproductive illness accounts for one third of the global burden of disease among women of reproductive age and 20% of the burden of disease among the general population. The need for reproductive health services is greatest among the poor. There are some 201 million women with unmet need for effective contraception. Meeting their needs, for an estimated annual cost of $3.9 billion, would avert some 52 million pregnancies each year and in turn prevent:

- 23 million unplanned births (72% reduction)
- 22 million induced abortions (64% reduction)
- 1.4 million infant deaths
- 142,000 pregnancy related-deaths (including 53,000 from unsafe abortions)

Additionally, 505,000 children would not lose their mothers to pregnancy related-deaths.

Investment in reproductive health services contributes to economic growth, societal and gender equity, and democratic governance. Unintended pregnancies, HIV, and other STIs strike men and women as they are entering their more productive years. Better health will result in reductions in public expenditures on education, health care, and social services, and thereby contribute to economic growth. By enabling young women to delay childbearing until they finish their education, reproductive health services offer women the opportunity to contribute to the country's development. On the other hand, failure to invest now in preventive services raises the future cost of meeting basic health care needs.

Providing contraceptive supplies and services to more than 200 million women around the world would cost $3.9 billion per year. More than 75% of spending on sexual and reproductive health care is shouldered by individuals, governments, and nongovernment organizations in developing counties. Wealthy nations are expected to cover one third of the cost, based on the proportions established at the 1994 International Conference on Population and Development at Cairo, Egypt. In 2000, developed countries provided less than 50% of what they had pledged.

According to the London-based humanitarian agency OXFAM, aid budgets in general have dwindled in the past 30 years. In the report, Paying the Price, the British aid agency said countries like the United States, Germany, and Japan had reneged on pledges made in 1970 to make available 0.7% of their gross national income (GNI) in aid. As a result, the aid budgets of rich nations were half what they were in 1960. OXFAM said that US aid was giving just 0.14% of GNI in aid. Much aid from the European Union arrived a year late, and Japan has cut its aid budget. Thirty percent of aid money is tied to an obligation to buy goods and services from the donor country. The situation becomes heartrending, because poor countries have to pay $100 million a day in debt repayments to institutions run by wealthy countries. The Philippines alone spends 10.9% of its gross domestic product (GDP) in debt servicing; in contrast, the expenditure for health is 1.6% of GDP. This is money that developing nations can put back into education, health and development programs [53].

In the end, providing contraceptive information and services to adolescents in developing countries has to be achieved in the context of gender equality, poverty alleviation, political will, and a just relationship between the have and have-not nations Societies from both ends of the economic spectrum have the ethical obligation to protect, enable, and empower young people as they negotiate the risks of adolescence. Wealthy nations should not hesitate to invest in the reproductive health of close to 1 billion youth in developing countries, because their sheer numbers will determine the demographics, economic development, health, and well-being, not only of their own countries and regions, but of the world also.

References

[1] United Nations. The world's women 2000: trends and statistics. New York: United Nations; 2000.

[2] United Nations Population Fund. Fast facts: young people and demographic trends. New York: UNFPA; 2000.

[3] Boyd A. The world's youth 2000. Washington (DC): Population Reference Bureau; 2000.

[4] Mehta S, Groenen R, Roque F. Adolescents in changing times: issues and perspectives for adolescent reproductive health in the ESCAP region [series no.153]. In: UNPFA report of the high-level meeting to review the implementation of the Program of Action of the International Conference on Population and Development and the Bali declaration on population and sustainable development. Bangkok (Thailand): 1998.

[5] Advocates for Youth. The sexual and reproductive health of youth: a global snapshot. Washington (DC): Advocates for Youth; 2003.

[6] Alan Guttmacher Institute. Into a new world: young women's sexual and reproductive lives. New York: The Alan Guttmacher Institute; 1998.

[7] Pachauri S, Santhya KG. Reproductive choices for Asian adolescents: a focus on contraceptive behavior. Int Fam Plann Perspect 2002;28(4):186–95 [http://www.agi-usa.org/pubs/journals/2818602.pdf].

[8] Henshaw S, Singh S, Haas T. The incidence of abortion worldwide. Fam Plann Perspect 1999; 25:S30–8.

[9] Population Action International. A world of difference: sexual and reproductive health and risks. Washington (DC): Population Action International; 2001.

[10] United Nations Population Fund. Fast facts: fistula and reproductive health. New York: UNFPA; 2004.

[11] United Nations Population Fund. State of world population 2003: HIV/AIDS and adolescents. New York: UNFPA; 2004.

[12] World Health Organization. Improving access to quality care in fertility planning: medical eligibility to contraceptive use. 3rd edition. Geneva (Switzerland): World Health Organization; 2004.

[13] American Academy of Pediatrics. Committee on adolescence. Contraception and adolescents. Pediatrics 1999;104:1161–6.

[14] National Statistics Office. Census of housing and population. Manila (Philippines): National Statistics Office; 2000.

[15] United Nations Population Fund. State of world population 2003. Monitoring ICPD goals: selected indicators. New York: UNFPA; 2003.

[16] United Nations Population Fund. Population and reproductive health country profile. New York: UNFPA; 2004.

[17] United Nations Population Fund. State of World Population 2003: gender inequality and reproductive health. New York: UNFPA; 2003.

[18] Brown AD, et al. Sexual relations among young people in developing countries: evidence from WHO case studies. Geneva (Switzerland): World Health Organization; 2000.

[19] Zablan ZC. Filipino youth's views on premarital sex and unmarried parenthood. Quezon City, (Philippines): University of the Philippines Population Institute; 1995.

[20] Raymundo CM, Cruz GT. Youth sex and risk behavior in the Philippines. Quezon City (Philippines): University of the Philippines Population Institute and Demographic Research and Development Foundation; Inc.; 2002.

[21] Jejeebhoy SJ, Bott S. Nonconsensual sexual experiences of young people: a review of the evidence for developing countries. South and East Asian regional working paper series number16. New Delhi (India): Population Council; 2003.

[22] Rani M, Lule E. Exploring the socio–economic dimension of adolescent reproductive health: a multi-country analysis. Inter Fam Plann Perspect 2004;30(3):110–7.

[23] Gueye M, Castle S, Konaté MK. Timing of first sex among Malian adolescents: implications for contraception. Inter Fam Plann Perspect 2001;27(2):56–62.

[24] Varga CA, Zosa-Feranil I. Adolescent reproductive health in the Philippines: status, policies, programs and issues. Philippines: Policy and US Agency for International Development. Washington (DC): (USAID); 2003.

[25] Raymundo CM, Xenos P, Domingo LJ. Adolescent sexuality in the Philippines. Quezon City (Philippines): University of the Philippines Population Institute and Office of the Vice Chancellor for Research and Development; 1999.

[26] United Nations Population Fund. Technical report: contraceptive requirements and logistics management needs in the Philippines. Manila (Philippines): United Nations Population Fund; 2002.

[27] United Nations Population Fund. State of world population 2004: reproductive health and family planning. New York: UNFPA; 2004.

[28] Best K. Why do people change methods? Family Health International. Available at: www.fhi.org/en/RH/Pubs/Network/v19_4/why_change.htm. Accessed June 28, 2005.

[29] Goody WR, Billy OG, Klepinger DH. Contraceptive switching in the United States. Perspect Sex Reprod Health 2002;34(3):135–45.

[30] Emans SJ. Contraception. In: Emans SJ, Laufer MR, Goldstein DP, editors. Pediatric and adolescent gynecology. Philadelphia: Lippincott Williams & Wilkins; 1998. p. 611–74.

[31] Department of Economics and Social Affairs Population Division. Contraceptive use according to women's marital status. Levels and trends of contraceptive use as assessed in 1998. New York: United Nations Publications; 2001. p. 91–103.

[32] Raymundo CM, Zablan ZC, Cabigon JV, et al. Unsafe abortion in the Philippines. Quezon City (Philippines): Demographic Research and Development Foundation, Inc. and the University of the Philippines Office of the Vice Chancellor for Research and Development; 2001.

[33] Commission on Population. ICPD at 10: Putting people first. Country report, Philippines. Mandaluyong City, (Philippines): POPCOM; 2004.

[34] Cheng TL, Savageu JA, Sattler AL, et al. Confidentiality in health care: a survey of knowledge, perceptions and attitudes among high school students. JAMA 1993;269(11):1404–7.

[35] Society for Adolescent Medicine. Confidential health services for adolescents: position paper. J Adolesc Health 2004;35(1):1–8.

[36] Solis PB. Medical jurisprudence. Manila (Philippines): RP Garcia Publishing Co.; 1988.

[37] English A. Understanding legal aspects of care. In: Neinstein LS, editor. Adolescent health care: a practical guide. 3rd edition. Baltimore (MD): Williams and Wilkins; 1996. p. 150–61.

[38] Montebon-Auxilio M, Villarmina S, Valeros E. NGOs debunk Catholic Church's claim that HB 4110 is proabortion. Available at: http://www.cyberdyaryo.com/features/f2003_0103_01.htm. Accessed June 28, 2005.

[39] Gastardo-Conaco MC, Jimenez MC, Billedo CJF. Filipino adolescents in changing times.

Quezon City (Philippines): University of the Philippines—Center for Women's Studies and Philippine Center for Population and Development; 2003.

[40] Tan ML, Batangan MTU, Cabado-Espanola H. Love and desire: young Filipinos and sexual risk. Quezon City (Philippines): University of the Philippines—Center for Women's Studies and the Ford Foundation; 2001.

[41] United Nations Population Fund. ICPD and MDG follow-up. ICPD: program of action, para. 7.43. New York: UNFPA; 2004.

[42] United Nations Population Fund. State of world population 2003: Promoting healthier behavior. New York: UNFPA; 2004.

[43] Commission on Population. State of the Philippine population report, 2nd issue. Pinoy youth: making choices, building voices. Mandaluyong City (Philippines): POPCOM; 2004.

[44] Society for Adolescent Medicine. Access to health care for adolescents and young adults: position paper. J Adolesc Health 1992;13:162–70.

[45] Society for Adolescent Medicine. School-based clinics: position paper. J Adolesc Health 2001; 29:448–50.

[46] Stevens C. In focus: reaching marginalized youth. Washington (DC): Pathfinders International; 1999.

[47] Pathfinders International. End of program report: advancing young adults' reproductive health: actions for the next decade. Washington (DC): Pathfinders International; 2001.

[48] Goodkind D, Anh PT. Reasons for rising condom use in Vietnam. Fam Plann Perspect 1997;23(4):173–8.

[49] DKT. Available at: www.dktinternational.org/philippines.htm. Accessed June 28, 2005.

[50] Mayhew S. Donor dealings: the impact of international donor aid on sexual and reproductive health services. Fam Plann Perspect 2002;28(4):220–4.

[51] Joint United Nations Programme on HIV/AIDS (UNAIDS). Executive Summary: 2004 repost on the global AIDS epidemic. New York: UNAIDS; 2004.

[52] Singh S, Darroch J, Vlassoff M, et al. Adding it up: the benefits of investing in sexual and reproductive health care. New York: The Alan Guttmacher Institute; 2004.

[53] Oxfam International. Paying the price: why rich countries must invest now in a war on poverty. Oxford (UK): Oxfam International; 2005.

ELSEVIER
SAUNDERS

Adolesc Med 16 (2005) 665–674

ADOLESCENT
MEDICINE
CLINICS

Practical Approaches to Prescribing Contraception in the Office Setting

Kristi Morgan Mulchahey, MD

Atlanta Gyn Associates, 2550 Windy Hill Road, Suite 115, Marietta, GA 30067, USA

Many adolescents will not seek contraceptive services until well after their first sexual intercourse [1]. Most adolescents do not seek contraceptive services until they have been sexually active for 6 months, yet 50% of adolescents will conceive within these first 6 months of unprotected intercourse [2,3]. In other words, many sexually active adolescents will be not seek care until it is too late. Initial access to care becomes crucial for preventing unintended adolescent pregnancy [4].

Early (12–14 years) and often middle (15–17 years) adolescents, are concrete thinkers; their inability to think abstractly limits their ability to make decisions and choices for future benefit. The use of all types of contraceptives requires some advance planning. This may become a barrier in delivering care to early and middle adolescents. To plan in advance requires acknowledging that sexual activity may occur in the near future. Many adolescents describe being swept away and not having planned intercourse.

Concrete thinkers also may have difficulty acknowledging the possibility of pregnancy. For example, early adolescents may admit that they are sexually active and comprehend the fact that sexual activity may produce a pregnancy, but they may be unable to acknowledge that they could become pregnant through unprotected intercourse. Understanding of personal vulnerability requires knowledge that an action taken now could produce a consequence in the future. Prevention of pregnancy also requires decisions and choices now to prevent an unforeseen event in the future.

Even older adolescents with a growing ability for abstract thinking may have ambivalence about the rightness or wrongness of their decision to be sexually

E-mail address: oaktrdr@aol.com

1547-3368/05/$ – see front matter © 2005 Elsevier Inc. All rights reserved.
doi:10.1016/j.admecli.2005.05.004
adolescent.theclinics.com

active. Sometimes, this ambivalence translates into poor contraceptive practices. Planning a contraceptive method implies that they have made an active
choice to be sexually active [5].

Barriers to care

The unique developmental tasks of adolescence may pose barriers to care
for contraceptive services. Encouraging abstinence (both primary and secondary)
while providing for contraceptive needs can be a difficult balance to achieve.
There are also other barriers to care for the adolescent that must be overcome.
For many adolescents, physical access to care is difficult. Teens may not know
where services are provided and how to find services at lower cost. Clinics or
offices without after-school appointments limit care. More school systems are
imposing penalties for absences, even those excused for a medical visit. Clinic/
office locations inconvenient to public transportation also limit care. The early to
middle adolescent may not be driving and may have to depend upon a parent
for transportation.

Language may be a barrier in an increasingly multicultural society. There
may be cultural barriers that make access to care especially difficult for first-
generation adolescents and their immigrant parents.

Concerns about confidentiality may stop some teens from seeking reproductive health services. Many studies have demonstrated that confidential treatment
encourages teens to seek contraceptive services earlier after sexual debut [10].
Confidential care should encourage family communication while acknowledging that many adolescents would not seek care if it were not confidential [11,12].
If confidentiality is not discussed early with the parents and teen, fear of anger
from parents toward the provider may interfere with provision of services.

Many adolescents feel that they cannot discuss issues of sexuality with their
parents [9]. Although confidential care should be available to all adolescents
for sexual health needs, not knowing how to discuss issues of sexuality with a
parent also can be a barrier to care. Many teens want to discuss their sexuality
with parents, but both parents and teens are equipped poorly to begin the conversation. Embarrassment, fear of punishment, or fear of disappointing parents
are all barriers. Being an askable parent is not a trait that comes automatically
with the addition of a new child to the family. Parents will bring to this experience their own feeling about their sexuality, especially sexual decisions that
they made during their own adolescence.

Paying for the services may pose another challenge, especially if the teen is
insured by a third party payer provided through a parent. Managed care and third
party payers add an additional level of concerns about confidentiality [6]. Confidentiality becomes an especially difficult issue for adolescents covered by
managed care plans where the parents are the primary insured individuals. Some
teens may be covered by health insurance provided by a noncustodial parent in
the event of divorce. These situations present a challenge for both the teen and the

care provider. Adolescents may not be aware of lower cost sources of care including school-based clinics, organizations such as Planned Parenthood, and family planning services available through their county health department. Those with Medicaid coverage may not realize that confidential family planning services are available.

Teens also may be reluctant to bring questions and concerns about sexual health to their pediatric health care providers. Some offices may be very child-friendly but not welcoming for adolescents and young adults. Some of the same barriers experienced with parents may be present again with the pediatrician as a parental authority figure. Physicians are also constrained by time, training, or ambivalence about providing contraceptives for teens. Spending time alone with the teen during each routine physical exam places additional stress on an already tight schedule in most offices [7]. Some pediatric care providers are not comfortable with providing pelvic exams in the office and are not aware that a pelvic exam is not essential before contraceptives are prescribed. Screening for sexually transmitted infection (STI) may be performed with new nucleic acid amplification-based technologies from a first voided urine sample.

Often teens have misconceptions regarding the efficacy and safety of contraceptive methods. There are many misconceptions about the safety of hormonal contraception among teenagers. Unfounded fears often include weight gain, acne, future infertility, and risk of cancer. The health benefits of hormonal contraception are underestimated, and the risks overestimated. Incorrect information often is perpetuated by the teen's peer group. These unfounded fears also may be shared by parents, especially concerns that hormonal contraception is dangerous for the younger adolescent. Parents often worry that hormonal contraceptive methods prescribed for medical indications will increase the possibility of sexual activity in their teen even though this has been proven not to be true.

Fear of a pelvic exam may stop some teens from requesting contraceptive services. There is much misinformation among adolescents about this procedure and fear of the examination itself. Most teens are not aware that hormonal methods of contraception may be prescribed without a pelvic exam [8].

A history of childhood sexual abuse or sexual assault also plays a role in adolescent sexual decision making. Several studies have noted that an earlier onset of sexual activity may be especially problematic with the early adolescent whose abstract thinking and advance planning skills may be limited. Sexual assault is common among adolescent girls and is often not identified by the girl herself as assault. The fear and shame associated with the trauma may prevent the girl from seeking reproductive health care services.

Practical pointers of counseling

In an ideal setting, all children would have easy access to a known, trusted, and approachable clinician. That clinician would have an effective and trusting partnership with the parents that began before adolescence, and issues of communication and confidentiality would be a routine part of anticipatory guidance. This formula would provide the best sexual health care for the adolescent. Unfortunately, as families are more mobile, care providers change frequently with a change in insurance status, and a growing number of adolescents are uninsured or underinsured, this ideal setting may be more the exception than the rule.

The best counseling for good sexual decision making and effective contraceptive use begins before the onset of sexual activity. Young adolescents should have access to accurate information about the risks of adolescent pregnancy, STIs, and strategies to reduce both, including abstinence. This involves a multidisciplinary approach with family, medical provider, school, and faith community.

Given the typical adolescent delay in seeking contraceptive services, effective contraceptive strategies need to be introduced before the onset of sexual activity. Teens need to be provided information regarding contraceptive methods during routine well adolescent exams. Effective strategies in the pediatric office can include written take-home material in waiting rooms, exam rooms, and restrooms. The material should be attractive and reading level appropriate. Posters, booklets, and other materials can be placed in restrooms where teens may read them in private. Providing early adolescents and their parents information together may encourage conversations at home. Explaining guidelines for confidential treatment of adolescent sexual health concerns is much easier when done before the need arises.

Teens also can be encouraged to share the information with peers who may be sexually active. Provide teens with several copies of information about the safety and efficacy of contraceptives and encourage them to leave them behind at school, movie theaters, malls, or on the bus. Adolescents often look to their peers for sexual information and can be encouraged to be a source of accurate information. Virginal teens can help dispel myths regarding the safety of contraception and help share information about access to care from school-based clinics, Planned Parenthood, and pubic health department clinics. Physicians who are reluctant to spend valuable counseling time in the office with those teens who are not sexually active should remember that they may be equipping an informal peer counselor [13].

The next step in effective counseling is availability. Barriers to availability can be addressed on a community level with school-based clinics, support of public health clinics, and effective sexuality education in the school that includes accurate contraceptive information. Health care providers still are viewed as community resources and may have a positive impact on community decisions if they take the time to become involved. Resources are available from the American College of Obstetricians and Gynecologists (ACOG) to assist in community education. The Adolescent Sexuality Tool Kit from ACOG contains helpful resources for practitioners to use in the office and community (www.acog.org).

In the office setting, barriers to care also need to be addressed. There are many ways that the office/clinic environment can be modified to encourage effective counseling. An environment that is welcoming to the adolescent may include a waiting space or area for teens. Publications of interest to teens including reading material about contraception may be provided. Some offices have found after-school appointments helpful. Office/clinic support staff who enjoy adolescents, who have a good understanding of the world of the adolescent, and who are trained in effective counseling strategies may increase compliance. Support staff should be nonjudgmental in their interactions with teens. All clinicians should be self-aware about their attitudes and judgments that can be communicated unintentionally to the teen seeking contraceptive services. Phone support availability for questions and problems has been found to be helpful [14]. Communication by E-mail also can be helpful when done properly.

Effective contraceptive use by the adolescent begins with anticipatory guidance from the care provider about common traps that may lead the adolescent to discontinue use or use a method incorrectly [15].

The teen should be actively involved in the choice of contraceptive method. For the average healthy teen, a hormonal method coupled with condom use is often the best choice. It is helpful, however, to talk through the process of choosing a method to allow the teen to be an active participant. The teen's active involvement in the selection process will help foster a sense of ownership of the method. There are various materials available to assist in the process. Most patients will retain only a small percentage of information provided during an office visit [16]. Written material to take home often is used, although some teens will be reluctant to take home written materials for fear of loss of confidentiality. There are a growing number of Web sites (www.aware.com among others) providing accurate and age-appropriate information for teens about contraceptive choices. Many of these sites are interactive, and some even allow questions about sexuality and contraception to be posted and answered by experts in the field. Adolescent patients all learn differently. Written materials may be helpful for some; audio or visual teaching tapes may help others. Seeing and holding a package of pills or a condom is valuable for some teens. The availability of pharmaceutical samples has been demonstrated to be an important tool in increasing compliance [17].

Teenagers often overestimate the dangers of oral contraceptives. This fear may lead to discontinuation when minor adverse effects develop [18]. It is important that the rarity of serious adverse effects be addressed. It is also important to mention the myths of pill use, such as fears of infertility or cancer. The common adjustment adverse effects, such as mild headaches, breakthrough bleeding, and occasional bloating should be discussed, so they will not be frightening to patients. It is especially helpful to advise teens starting oral contraceptives that they should contact the provider before making the decision to discontinue their pills. It is important to discuss the possibility of an occasional amenorrheic cycle with oral contraceptives. The absence of a withdrawal period frightens many teens, often leading to discontinuation of the method. On the other hand, teens should be instructed to come in for a pregnancy test if they do miss a period, because use of contraceptives can be imperfect. Sometimes teens will experience breakthrough bleeding and decide that they should stop their pills to allow a period. Both situations can result in unintended pregnancies [19].

Prescribing practices need to take cost of the method into account to increase compliance. Discussing the cost of the method and how the teen will pay for the prescription is important. Adolescents are less knowledgeable than most adults about costs, the use of insurance prescription coverage, and the available of lower cost contraceptives from the health department or agencies. Many teenagers have never filled a prescription and may have no idea what to do with the small piece of paper they are given in the office. This presents a valuable teaching opportunity to explain how prescriptions are filled, how they are paid for, and the importance of planning ahead. Providing the patient with a sample package of pills, patches, or a vaginal ring just in case they cannot get to the pharmacy is often helpful. Day one of cycle starts or quick starts of cyclic oral contraceptives may be more practical than Sunday starts [20]. Most clinics and providers are not available on Sundays if a prescription needs refilling; not all pharmacies and most agencies are not open for dispensing or questions on weekends.

Increasing compliance with condom use requires careful instruction in proper use but also requires negotiation skills with a partner, and the adolescent may not possess these skills. It may be helpful to practice a dialog between the teen and her partner. There are several commercial booklets available to allow teens to practice these conversations. Younger adolescents at high risk for STIs or pregnancy may not be able to learn these skills; sometimes it can be helpful to encourage the adolescent to blame her care provider for the need to use condoms. "If you don't want to use condoms, my doctor/nurse said that you would have to come and talk to them" may be a helpful statement for the adolescent to learn.

Many adolescents find the daily dosing of oral contraceptives difficult, and this can result in breakthrough bleeding. The common teachings of "take your pill at bedtime" or "take your pill when you brush your teeth at bedtime" are not effective in adolescents who often have different weekend and weekday schedules. Placing a reminder note on the bathroom mirror will not work if the teen's parents are not aware of her contraceptive use. One solution that often works is encouraging the teen to wear an inexpensive sports watch with the alarm set for the daily time the pill needs to be taken. If the teen will keep her pills in her purse or backpack, she can be reminded by the alarm on the watch to stay on schedule with her pills. Using a different delivery system, such as a vaginal contraceptive ring or a contraceptive transdermal patch, may also help with these compliance problems.

There are clinical situations that present special opportunities for counseling to increase contraceptive compliance. The teen who presents for pregnancy testing and has a negative pregnancy test will be relieved; this can be an important moment to re-evaluate her contraceptive method, her compliance, and adverse effects of the method. Teens taking oral contraceptives can be reminded of proper pill use in the face of a missed withdrawal bleed, breakthrough bleeding, or missed pills. Pregnancy testing is often done on a walk-in basis by clinic support staff. These individuals should have training to recognize these teachable moments and take advantage of that negative pregnancy test and a teen who is often receptive to teaching at that moment of relief.

Abortion counseling (both before and after the procedure) is another opportunity to discuss prevention of future unintended pregnancies. This should be provided by the clinic providing the termination services, but this does not always happen. Contraceptive counseling should begin at the time diagnosis of the unintended pregnancy, which is often in the primary clinician's office. It should be a part of all postabortal follow-up visits. Spontaneous abortion is also frequent in the adolescent population. This may be the first contact of the adolescent girl with the health care system, and compliance with follow-up visits may be poor. This contact is an opportunity that should not be missed.

Adolescents are very likely to resume sexual activity soon after delivery of a baby. The third trimester of pregnancy is an optimal time to discuss postpartum contraceptives with the pregnant adolescent. This should be discussed again before discharge from the hospital. No teen should leave the hospital without a clear plan for prevention of unintended pregnancy.

Parental involvement/confidentiality

In the perfect world, parents, schools, and health care professionals would work together to provide information about pregnancy and STI prevention as a part of sexuality education before sexual debut. Unfortunately, this does not happen often. In fact, some adolescents feel that they cannot discuss issues of contraception with their parents. Many sexually active teens worry about anger, disappointment, or shame from their parents [21]. These concerns may interfere with their ability of obtain and use effective contraception [22]. This has led most states to enact legislation or health care policy to allow teens to receive confidential family planning services.

Allowing teens to give their own consent for health care and counseling services relating to pregnancy prevention/diagnosis/treatment, STI diagnosis/treatment, and termination of pregnancy is permitted in most states. Individual states have enacted legislation to restrict teen access to some services, especially abortion services, without parental consent. Each state has different legal requirements for adolescents to provide informed consent, and it is the responsibility of each practitioner to have a clear understanding of the laws and requirements of the state in which he or she practices. ACOG and the American Academy of Pediatrics have position papers in favor of teen access to confidential family planning services [23].

Although laws vary from state to state, there are several legal and ethical principles that apply in all jurisdictions. Traditionally, parents make all decisions about the lives of their minor children, including health care decisions and informed consent, and are responsible financially for their children's health care. The courts have recognized, however, that there are circumstances where requiring parental consent for treatment would interfere with the ability of the adolescent to obtain necessary medical treatment. In general, these circumstances involve family abuse or sensitive subjects (related to sexual activity or substance abuse). Emancipated minors are able to provide their own consent for medical treatment; generally, emancipated minors are those who are married, living separate from parents without financial support, or in the military.

Consent for sensitive services, especially contraceptive-, pregnancy-, and STI-related care, is different for each legal jurisdiction and generally determined on the state level. It is important that each clinician be familiar with the policies and laws of the state in which he or she practices. At present, provision of abortion services to adolescents is the most controversial. When parental notification is required by the state, there is usually a provision for judicial bypass, where the court may authorize the adolescent to give her own consent [24–26].

For the adolescent to provide her own consent, the basic principles of informed consent must be met. Specifically, the patient must understand the diagnosis, risks, and benefits of treatment, alternative choices, and risks of not undergoing the recommended treatment. In some states, it is up to the clinician to determine the degree of understanding of the adolescent. Studies have shown that most adolescents are capable of giving informed consent for medical decisions [27]. In clinical settings where parents are responsible for informed consent (eg, before surgical procedures), there is still benefit in involving the adolescent in the process. This may increase compliance by the adolescent and is good preparation for adulthood [28,29].

Confidentiality of written and verbal communication between the clinician and the patient also is protected under the law. This extends to the adolescent in situations where they are able to provide their own informed consent for care. Exceptions to this rule would include reportable abuse, serious danger of self-harm or harm to others, and certain reportable STIs. The clinician has an ethical obligation to disclose that information to the patient at the onset of care.

The clinician must learn to walk a fine line between encouraging productive parental involvement and making sure that teens receive the reproductive health care they need. Anticipatory guidance for parents should include a discussion of adolescent confidentiality, preferably before a crisis develops. Clinicians should discuss the subject of confidentiality with parents and teens and assist in developing a good working relationship between the teen, parent, and clinician. Clinicians should support good teen–parent communication about all subjects, including those related to sexuality.

In summary, providing teens with age appropriate contraceptive services requires a clinician who has a good understanding the many facets of the life of the teen that will impact their contraceptive choices and compliance. The clinician should strive to foster good parent–teen communication, while at the same time maintaining confidentiality. A good understanding of home, school, and community environments will facilitate pregnancy prevention. All interactions with teens need to be approached with a good understanding of the pertinent developmental issues and an understanding of various education strategies to increase compliance. A team approach between family, school, community, and health care professional will give each adolescent the best chance for healthy sexual decision making.

References

[1] Manning WD, Longmore MA, Giordano PC. The relationship context of contraceptive use at first intercourse. Fam Plann Perspect 2000;32(3):104–10.

[2] Johnson R. Race, adolescent contraceptive choice, and pregnancy at presentation to a family planning clinic. Obstet Gynecol 2002;100(1):174.

[3] Santelli JS, Lindberg LD, Abma J, et al. Adolescent sexual behavior: estimates and trends from four nationally representative surveys. Fam Plann Perspect 2000;32(4):156–65.

[4] Manlove J, Ryan S, Franzetta K. Patterns of contraceptive use within teenagers' first sexual relationships. Perspect Sex Reprod Health 2003;35(6):246–55.

[5] Lagana L. Psychosocial correlates of contraceptive practices during late adolescence. Adolescence 1999;34(135):463–82.

[6] Sugerman S, Halfon N, Fink A, et al. Family planning clinic patients: their usual health care providers, insurance status, and implications for managed care. J Adolesc Health 2000;27(1): 25–33.

[7] Merzel CR, Vandevanter NI, Middlestadt S, et al. Attitudinal and contextual factors association with discussion of sexual issues during adolescent health visits. J Adolesc Health 2004;35(2): 108–15.

[8] Stewart FH, Harper CC, Ellertson CE, et al. Clinical breast and pelvic exam requirements for hormonal contraception: current practice vs evidence. JAMA 2001;285(17):2232–9.

[9] Jaccard J, Dittus PJ. Adolescent perceptions of maternal approval of birth control and sexual risk behavior. Am J Public Health 2000;90(9):1426–30.

[10] Brindis CD, Llewelyn L, Marie K, et al. Meeting the reproductive health care needs of adolescents: California's family planning access, care, and treatment program. J Adolesc Health 2003;32:79–80.

[11] Council on Scientific Affairs. Confidential health services for adolescents. JAMA 1993;269: 1420–4.

[12] Reddy DM, Fleming R, Swain C. Effects of mandatory parental notification on adolescent girls' use of sexual health care services. JAMA 2002;288(6):710–4.

[13] Yanda K. Teenagers educating teenagers about reproductive health and their rights to confidential care. Fam Plann Perspect 2000;32(5):256–7.

[14] Parker BL. Teen-friendly services: advocates for successful teen contraception. N J Med 2000;97(2):41–4.

[15] Zibners A, Cromer BA, Hayes J. Comparison of continuation rates for hormonal contraception among adolescents. J Pediatr Adolesc Gynecol 1999;12(2):90–4.

[16] Issacs JN, Crenin MD. Miscommunication between healthcare providers and patients may results in unplanned pregnancies. Contraception 2003;68(5):373–6.

[17] Zink T, Rosenthal S. The use of oral contraceptive pharmaceutical sample packs by adolescent health care providers. J Pediatr Adolesc Gynecol 2000;12(3):129–33.

[18] Longmore MA, Manning WD, Giordano PC, et al. Contraceptive self-efficacy; does it influence adolescents' contraceptive use? J Health Soc Behav 2003;44(1):45–60.

[19] Johnston-Robledo I, Ball M, Lauta K, et al. To bleed or not to bleed: young women's attitudes toward menstrual suppression. Women Health 2003;38(3):59–75.

[20] Lara-Torre E, Schroeder B. Adolescent compliance and side effects with Quick Start initiation of oral contraceptive pills. Contraception 2002;66(2):81–5.

[21] Miller BD. Family influences of adolescent sexual and contraceptive behavior. J Sex Res 2002;39(1):22–6.

[22] Jones RK, Soonstra H. Confidential reproductive health services for minors: the potential impact of mandated parental involvement for contraception. Perspect Sex Reprod Health 2004;36(5): 182–91.

[23] American College of Obstetrics and Gynecology. ACOG technical bulletin. The adolescent obstetric–gynecologic patient. Washington (DC): American College of Obstetrics and Gynecology; 1990.

[24] English A, Simmons PS. Legal issues in reproductive health care for adolescents. Adolesc Med 1999;10(2):181–94.

[25] English A. The health of adolescent girls: does the law support it? Curr Womens Health Rep 2002;2(6):442–9.

[26] English A. Reproductive health services for adolescent: critical legal issues. Obstet Gynecol Clin North Am 2000;27(1):195–221.

[27] Gittler J, Quigley-Rick M, Saks MJ. Adolescent health care decision making: the law and public policy. Washington (DC): Carnegie Council on Adolescent Development; 1990.

[28] Cook R, Dickens BM. Recognizing adolescents' evolving capacities to exercise choice in reproductive healthcare. Int J Gynaecol Obstet 2000;70(1):13–21.

[29] Saul R. Teen pregnancy: progress meets politics. Guttmacher Rep Public Policy 1999;2(3):6–9.

ELSEVIER
SAUNDERS

ADOLESCENT
MEDICINE
CLINICS

Adolesc Med 16 (2005) 675–676

Erratum

Erratum to "Video Killed the Radio Star: The Effects of Music Videos on Adolescent Health" [Adolesc Med 16 (2) (2005) 371–393]

Sarah L. Ashby, MD[a], Michael Rich, MD, MPH[b],*

[a]Department of Pediatrics, University of Wisconsin–Madison, 777 South Mills Street, Madison, WI 53715, USA
[b]Center on Media and Child Health, Division of Adolescent/Young Adult Medicine, Children's Hospital Boston, 300 Longwood Avenue, Boston, MA 02115, USA

In the June 2005 issue "Adolescents and the Media," in the article "Video Killed the Radio Star: The Effects of Music Videos on Adolescent Health" by Sarah L. Ashby and colleagues, the incorrect version of some of the references were published. The corrected references appear below and the corrected article can be found online at www.adolescent.theclinics.com.

References

[6] Rich M. Boy, mediated: effects of entertainment media on male adolescent health. In: Rosen DS, Rich M, editors. Adolescent medicine: state of the art reviews—the adolescent male. Philadelphia: Hanley & Belfus; 2003. p. 691–715.

[7] Strasburger VC, Wilson BJ. Children, adolescents and the media. Thousand Oaks (CA): Sage Publications; 2002.

[8] Brown JD, Witherspoon EM. The mass media and American adolescents' health. J Adolesc Health 2002;31:153–70.

[9] Villani S. Impact of media on children and adolescents: a 10-year review of the research. J Am Acad Child Adolesc Psychiatry 2001;40:392–401.

[10] Strasburger VC, Donnerstein E. Children, adolescents, and the media: issues and solutions. Pediatrics 1999;103:129–39.

Doi of original article title 10.1016/j.admecli.2005.02.001

* Corresponding author.

[11] Klein JD, Brown JD, Childers KW, et al. Adolescents' risky behavior and mass media use. Pediatrics 1993;92:24–31.

[12] Bushman BJ, Huesmann LR. Effects of televised violence on aggression. In: Singer DG, Singer JL, editors. Handbook of children and the media. Thousand Oaks (CA): Sage Publications; 2001. p. 223–54.

[13] Paik H, Comstock G. The effects of television violence on antisocial-behavior: a meta-analysis. Communic Res 1994;21:516–46.

[14] Hearold S. A synthesis of 1043 effects of television on social behavior. Public Communication and Behavior 1986;1:65–133.

[15] Andison F. TV violence and viewer aggressiveness: a cumulation of study results 1956–1976. Public Opin Q 1977;41:314–31.

[16] Brown JD, Walsh-Childers K, Steele JR. Sexual teens, sexual media: investigating media's influence on adolescent sexuality. Mahwah (NJ): Lawrence Erlbaum; 2002.

[17] Sargent JD, Dalton MA, Beach ML, et al. Viewing tobacco use in movies: does it shape attitudes that mediate adolescent smoking? Am J Prev Med 2002;22:137–45.

[18] Distefan J, Gilpin E, Sargent JD, et al. Do movie stars encourage adolescents to start smoking? Evidence from California. Prev Med 1999;28:1–11.

[19] Austin E, Knaus C. Predicting future risky behavior among those "too young" to drink as the result of advertising desirability. Presented at the Association for Education in Journalism and Mass Communication Meeting. Baltimore, Maryland, August 5–8, 1998.

[20] Austin E, Meili H. Effects of interpretations of televised alcohol portrayals on children's alcohol beliefs. J Broadcast Electr Media 1994;38:417–35.

[21] Connolly GM, Caswell S, Zhang JF, et al. Alcohol in the mass media and drinking by adolescents: a longitudinal study. Addiction 1994;89:1255–63.

[39] The Henry J. Kaiser Family Foundation. The 1996 Kaiser Family Foundation Survey on Teens and Sex: what they say teens today need to know, and who they listen to. Menlo Park (CA): The Henry J. Kaiser Family Foundation; 1996.

[41] The Henry J. Kaiser Family Foundation/Children Now. Talking with kids about tough issues: a national survey of parents and kids. Menlo Park (CA): The Henry J. Kaiser Family Foundation; 1999.

[44] Tapper J, Thorson E, Black D. Variations in music videos as a function of their musical genre. J Broadcast Electr Media 1994;38:103–13.

[48] Bauman KE, Botvin GJ, Botvin EM, et al. Normative expectations and the behavior of significant others: an integration of traditions in research on adolescents' cigarette smoking. Psychol Rep 1992;71:568–70.

[50] Seidman SA. An investigation of sex-role stereotyping in music videos. J Broadcast Electr Media 1992;36:209–16.

[55] Signorielli N, McLeod D, Healy E. Gender stereotypes in MTV commercials: the beat goes on. J Broadcast Electr Media 1994;38:91–101.

[63] Brown JD, Steele J. Sex and the mass media. Menlo Park (CA): The Henry J. Kaiser Family Foundation; 1995.

[99] Malamuth NM, Check JVP. The effects of mass media exposure on acceptance of violence against women: a field experiment. J Res Pers 1981;15:436–46.

[100] Malamuth NM, Briere J. Sexual violence in the media: indirect effects on aggression against women. J Soc Issues 1986;42:75–92.

[110] Scharrer E. Making a case for media literacy in the curriculum: outcomes and assessment. J Adolescent Adult Literacy 2002;46:354–8.

[111] Silverblatt A. Media literacy: keys to interpreting media messages. Westport (CT): Praeger; 2001.

[112] Hansen CH, Hansen RD. Rock music and antisocial behavior. Basic Appl Soc Psychol 1990; 11:357–69.

ELSEVIER
SAUNDERS

Adolesc Med 16 (2005) 677–691

ADOLESCENT
MEDICINE
CLINICS

Cumulative Index 2005

Note: Page numbers of article titles are in **boldface** type.

A

Abortifacients
    and herbal contraception, 609–610
    and pennyroyal, 610

Abortion counseling, 671

Abortion trends, 487

ABPM. See *Ambulatory blood pressure monitoring.*

ACE inhibitors. See *Angiotensin-converting enzyme inhibitors.*

Acne
    and oral contraceptive pills, 540–541

Acquired renal cystic disease, 127

Acute lymphocytic leukemia, 124

Acute renal failure, **1–9**
    exercise-associated, 114–115
    and NSAIDs, 115

Acute tubular necrosis
    and STDs, 49, 55

ADH. See *Antidiuretic hormone.*

Adolescent contraception
    and parental involvement, 671–672

Adolescent smoking
    and influence of the media, 346–350
    and link to favorite star smoking, 353–356
    and measuring media influence, 352–353
    and media literacy, 365
    and onset of tobacco use, 346
    and parenting style, 356–358
    and policy interventions, 358–363
    and role of the pediatrician/adolescent specialist, 365–366
    and the V-chip, 363–364

Adolescent urology, **215–227**

Adolescents, sex, and the media: ooooo, baby, baby—a Q & A, **269–288**

Adolescents and media literacy, **463–480**

Adolescents and media violence: six crucial issues for practitioners, **249–268**

Adolescents and the Internet, **413–426**

Adolescents' media diet pyramid, 258

Adolescents with proteinuria and/or the nephrotic syndrome, **163–172**

Advertising
    of alcohol, 333–338
    antitobacco, 364
    of birth control products, 278–281

Alcohol
    and the media, 327–339

Alcohol advertising, 333–338
    and effect on drinking beliefs and behaviors among youth, 334–335
    expenditures for, 333–336
    images in, 334
    restrictions on, 336–337

Alcohol in the media: content and effects on drinking beliefs and behaviors among youth, **327–343**

Alport syndrome
    and glomerulonephritis, 78–79

Ambulatory blood pressure monitoring, 22, 24, 26

Amphetamine abuse
    and nephrotoxicity, 40

Analgesic nephropathy, 31–32

Analgesics
    over-the-counter, 31–32

ANCA. See *Antineutrophil cytoplasmic autoantibody.*

Anemia
    and chronic kidney disease, 190–191
    and oral contraceptive pills, 542

1547-3368/05/$ – see front matter © 2005 Elsevier Inc. All rights reserved.
doi:10.1016/S1547-3368(05)00052-5   *adolescent.theclinics.com*

Angiotensin-converting enzyme inhibitors,
    24–26, 69, 72, 74
    and chronic kidney disease, 191–192
    and diabetic nephropathy, 179–180
    and glomerulonephritis, 69, 72, 74
    and hypertension, 24–26
    and nephrotic syndrome, 170

Anorexia
    and influence of the media, 293–296

Anti-GBM disease. See *Antiglomerular
    basement membrane disease.*

Antidiuretic hormone
    and hyponatremia, 114

Antiglomerular basement membrane disease
    and glomerulonephritis, 79

Antineutrophil cytoplasmic autoantibody
    and glomerulonephritis, 79–80

Antiotensin antagonists
    and treatment of STDs, 57–59

Antitobacco advertising
    in movies, 364

ARCD. See *Acquired renal cystic disease.*

ARF. See *Acute renal failure.*

ATN. See *Acute tubular necrosis.*

Autoimmune disease
    and contraception, 641

B

Bacteriuria
    and urinary tract infections, 153

Barrier and spermicidal contraceptives in
    adolescence, **495–515**

Bedwetting, 222–223

Benign breast disease
    and oral contraceptive pills, 541

Birt-Hogg-Dubé syndrome, 131

Birth control advertising
    and effect on teenage sexual activity,
        278–280
    network standards for, 281

Birth rates
    among U.S. teenagers, 485–488

Bladder dysfunction, 222–224
    and posterior urethral valves, 224
    and spina bifida, 223

Bladder stones, 87–107

Blood pressure, 6, 11–26
    definition of normal and abnormal,
        13–18
    and diabetic nephropathy, 177–178
    normative values, 14–17
    and obesity, 12–13

BMD. See *Bone mineral density.*

Body image
    adolescents' construction of, 290–291
    defined, 289–290
    and eating disorders, 293
    influence of music videos on, 376–377,
        385–386
    and influence of the family and
        peers, 295
    and the media, 280–281, 289–307
    content analyses, 298–300
    correlational studies, 300–301
    experimental studies, 301
    and interventions, 302–304
    qualitative research, 301–302
    research on, 298–302
    setting policy, 304–307
    negative, 292–294
    and obesity, 292–293

Body image and media use among adolescents,
    289–313

Bone marrow transplantation nephropathies, 141

Bone mineral density
    and depot medroxyprogesterone acetate,
        574–580

Breastfeeding
    and oral contraceptive pills, 544
    and progestin-only contraception, 543

Bulimia
    and influence of the media, 293–296

C

Cancer and the kidney, **121–148**

Candida albicans infection
    and urinary tract infections, 152

Cardiovascular disease
    and chronic kidney disease, 191–192
    and oral contraceptive pills, 546
    and progestin-only contraception,
        547–548, 560–564
    and proteinuria, 166

Cerebrovascular accidents
    and oral contraceptive pills, 518, 522

Cervical caps, 510–511
    advantages of, 511
    disadvantages of, 511

efficacy of, 511
proper use of, 511

Chinese herbs nephropathy, 33–34

Chlamydia trachomatis infection
and urinary tract infections, 151,
154, 156

Chronic kidney disease, 185–196
and ACE inhibitors, 191–192
and anemia, 190–191
and angiotensin receptor blockers, 192
and cardiovascular disease, 191–192
clinical consequences of, 187–196
and end-stage renal disease, 191,
195–196
epidemiology of, 186–187
and fluid, electrolyte, and acid-base
balance, 188–190
and glomerular filtration rate, 185–186,
189, 194
and growth, 193–194
and hypertension, 191–192
and metabolic bone disease, 192–193
and parathyroid hormone secretion, 193
psychosocial impact of, 194–195

Chronic kidney disease in adolescents,
185–199

Chronic renal insufficiency, 186, 189–193

Cisplatin
nephrotoxicity of, 138–139

CKD. See *Chronic kidney disease.*

Clq nephropathy
and glomerulonephritis, 77

CMV. See *Cytomegalovirus.*

Coca-Cola
and exclusive agreements with schools,
455–456

Cocaine abuse
and nephrotoxicity, 39

Cognitive Priming Theory
and media influence, 382

Colorectal cancer
and oral contraceptive pills, 540

Combined hormonal contraception, **517–537**
comparison of methods, 529
injectable, 533
medical eligibility criteria for, 524–526

Condoms
advantages of, 497–499, 502
in developing countries, 650
disadvantages of, 499, 502–503
efficacy of, 497–499, 501–502

female, 501–503
and latex allergy, 500
male, 489, 496–501
and prevention of STDs, 496, 498,
501–502
proper use of, 499, 503
troubleshooting, 500–501

Contraception
adolescent medical care for, 488–489
and autoimmune disease, 641
barrier and spermicidal, 495–512
and barriers to care, 666–667
for the chronically ill, 635–643
combined hormonal, 517–534
and confidentiality of medical care,
488–489, 666, 671–672
counseling adolescents about, 667–671
and cystic fibrosis, 639
in developing countries, 645–661
and effects on sexual behavior and risk,
491–492
emergency, 491, 555–556, 585–600,
627–628
and endocrine disorders, 637
and gastrointestinal illness, 639–640
and heart disease, 637–638
and hematologic and oncologic
problems, 640
hormonal, 489–491, 517–534
and immobility, 641
and inflammatory bowel disease, 639
male hormonal, 628–629
and mental retardation, 641–642
methods available to adolescents, 489–490
and neurological disorders, 636–637
and new products in development,
630–631
newer methods of, 490–491
oral, 489–491, 517–534
and other medications, 642
overview of, 485–492
prescribing in the office setting, 665–672
and pulmonary disease, 639
and renal disease, 638–639
and sickle cell disease, 640
and systemic lupus erythematosus, 641

Contraceptive choices for chronically ill
adolescents, **635–644**

Contraceptive issues of youth and adolescents
in developing countries: highlights from
the Philippines and other Asian countries,
645–663

Contraceptive research, 617–632

Contraceptive sponge, 506–507
efficacy of, 507
precautions for use of, 507
and prevention of STDs, 507

Contraceptive vaccines, 632

Cotton plant
    as a male antifertility agent, 611
    as a spermicidal agent, 610

Creatine use
    in adolescent athletes, 115
    and nephrotoxicity, 34–35

Creatinine clearance
    and kidney disease, 49–51

CRI. See Chronic renal insufficiency.

Cultivation Theory
    and media influence, 382

Current contraceptive research and develop-
    ment, **617–633**

CVA. See Cerebrovascular accidents.

Cystic fibrosis
    and contraception, 639

Cystinuria
    and urolithiasis, 102–103

Cystitis, 149–158
    treatment of, 156–158

Cytomegalovirus
    and kidney disease, 54
    and kidney transplantation, 206, 208

D

DASH. See Dietary Approaches to
    Stop Hypertension.

Deep vein thrombosis
    and progestin-only contraception,
        561–563

Depot medroxyprogesterone acetate, 543,
    553–554, 569–581, 625–626,
    636–642
    and bone mineral density, 574–578
    and contraception for chronically ill
        adolescents, 636–642
    via injection, 625–626
    and weight gain, 570–574

Depot medroxyprogesterone acetate:
    implications for weight status and bone
    mineral density in the adolescent female,
    569–584

Desensitization in adolescents
    and media violence, 257, 402–404, 476
    and violent video games, 402–404, 476

Developing countries
    barriers to contraception in, 653–655
    condom use in, 650

contraception in, 645–661
    contraceptive knowledge among
        adolescents in, 649–655
    expanding contraceptive options in,
        655–659
    gender inequality in, 648
    gender roles in, 648–649
    intrauterine devices in, 650–651
    oral contraceptive pills in, 651, 653
    poverty and reproductive health in, 649
    sexually transmitted diseases in,
        646–650, 652, 654–660
    socio-cultural milieu of adolescents in,
        648–649
    unmet contraceptive needs in, 655

Diabetes, 166–167, 173–182
    causes in adolescents, 173–174
    and glomerular structure, 178
    and progestin-only contraception, 564
    and proteinuria, 166–167

Diabetes mellitus and the kidney in
    adolescents, **173–184**

Diabetic nephropathy, 173–182
    and ACE inhibitors, 179–180
    and blood pressure, 177–181
    and end-stage renal disease,
        173–174, 181
    and glycemic control, 181
    history of, 174–175
    and lipid-lowering therapy, 179–180
    and metabolic control, 178–179
    and microalbuminuria, 176–177
    prevention and treatment of, 178–181
    and puberty, 175–176
    stages of, 174

Dialysis
    peritoneal, 7
    and renal failure, 6–7
    and STDs, 60–61

Diaphragms, 508–510
    advantages of, 509
    disadvantages of, 509
    efficacy of, 508–509
    and prevention of STDs, 509
    proper use of, 509–510

Dietary Approaches to Stop Hypertension, 23

DMPA. See Depot medroxyprogesterone acetate.

Drug abuse
    and nephrotoxicity, 36–40

Drug development process, 620–621

DVT. See Deep vein thrombosis.

Dysmenorrhea
    and oral contraceptive pills, 541–542

E

Eating disorders
  and influence of the media, 281–282,
    293–296

Ecstasy
  and nephrotoxicity, 40

Ectopic pregnancy
  and oral contraceptive pills, 541
  and progestin-only contraception, 543

Emergency contraception, 491, 555, **585–602**,
    627–628
  advance provision for, 597–599
  and adverse effects, 592–593
  and behavior change counseling,
    599–600
  complications of, 593–594
  efficacy of, 588–591
  failure rates of, 589–591
  and impact on sexual behavior,
    595–597
  indications for, 586
  and mechanism of action, 591–592
  with other methods of contraception,
    594–595
  products available for, 587–588

End-stage renal disease, 67, 72–74, 78–80,
    117, 127, 191, 195–196

Endometrial cancer
  and oral contraceptive pills, 540
  and progestin-only contraception, 543

Escherichia coli infection
  and urinary tract infections, 150,
    153, 157

ESRD. See *End-stage renal disease.*

Estrogen
  and emergency contraception,
    587–593
  and new developments in contraception,
    622–624
  and oral contraceptive pills, 520

ESWL. See *Extracorporeal shock
  wave lithotripsy.*

Extracorporeal shock wave lithotripsy
  and urolithiasis, 106–107, 219

F

Fear in adolescents
  and media violence, 255–257

Female condoms, 501–503

Fibroids
  and oral contraceptive pills, 542

Focal segmental glomerular sclerosis, 49–50,
    53–55, 59, 167–168
  and nephrotic syndrome, 167–168

FSGS. See *Focal segmental
  glomerular sclerosis.*

G

Gender inequality
  in developing countries, 648

Gender roles
  in developing countries, 648–649

Glomerular filtration rate
  and kidney disease, 49–51

Glomerulonephritis, **67–85**
  and ACE inhibitors, 69, 72, 74
  acute, 69–72
  and Alport syndrome, 78–79
  and antiglomerular basement membrane
    disease, 79
  and antineutrophil cytoplasmic
    autoantibody, 79–80
  chronic or persistent, 72–81
  and Clq nephropathy, 77
  diagnosis of, 68–69
  differential diagnoses of, 69
  and IgA nephropathy, 72–74
  membranoproliferative, 50, 54, 56–57,
    75–77
  and membranous nephropathy, 77–78
  pauci-immune, 80
  poststreptococcal acute, 70–72
  rapidly progressive, 70
  signs and symptoms of, 68
  and systemic lupus erythematosus,
    68–69, 76, 80–81
  treatment of, 69

Goodpasture's disease, 79

Gore, Tipper
  and music album advisory labels, 431

H

HAART. See *Highly active
  antiretroviral therapy.*

HBV. See *Hepatitis B virus.*

HCV. See *Hepatitis C virus.*

Headaches
  and oral contraceptive pills, 546

Heart disease
  and contraception, 637–638

Hematuria, 36, 111–113, 153, 229–238
    in adolescent athletes, 111–113
    and adolescent evaluation, 233–235
    causes and mechanisms of, 112
    differential diagnoses of, 232–233
    incidence and prevalence of, 231–232
    and laboratory and radiologic evaluation,
        235–237
    and natural medicines, 36
    and urinary tract infections, 153

Hematuria in adolescents, 229–239

Hemofiltration
    and renal failure, 7

Hemolytic uremic syndrome, 49–50, 54

Henoch-Schönlein purpura nephritis, 75

Hepatitis B virus
    and kidney disease, 45–46, 50, 54, 56,
        58, 61

Hepatitis C virus
    and kidney disease, 45–46, 50, 54, 56,
        58–59, 61

Hepatobiliary disease
    and progestin-only contraception, 564

Herbal contraception, 606–612
    and abortifaciens, 609–610
    and male antifertility herbs, 611–612
    and ovulation inhibition, 607–609
    and spermicidal agents, 610

Heroin abuse
    and HIV infection, 37, 39

Heroin-associated nephropathy, 36–37, 39

Highly active antiretroviral therapy
    and treatment of STDs, 53, 56–58,
        60–62

HIV-1–associated nephropathy, 51, 53–55,
        60–62

HIV infection. See Human immunodeficiency
    virus infection.

HIVAN. See HIV-1–associated nephropathy.

Hodgkin's disease, 124

Hormonal contraception, 489–491,
        517–534
    and extended cycle regimens,
        618–622
    historical perspective, 517–518
    inplants for, 626–627
    and low-dose formulations, 622
    for men, 628–629
    newer delivery methods of, 528–532
    recent and future trends in, 618–627

Hormonal contraception: noncontraceptive
    benefits and medical contraindications,
    539–551

Human immunodeficiency virus infection
    and heroin abuse, 37, 39
    and kidney disease, 45–47, 49–51,
        53–57, 59–62

HUS. See Hemolytic uremic syndrome.

Hydronephrosis, 216–218
    radiographic evaluation of, 217–218

Hypercalciuria
    and urolithiasis, 94–97

Hyperkalemia
    and renal failure, 5–6

Hypertension, 6, 11–26
    and ACE inhibitors, 24–26
    in adolescent athletes, 117
    and antihypertensive agents, 24–26
    causes in adolescents, 18–19
    and chronic kidney disease, 191–192
    diagnosis of, 19–22
    and diet, 23
    and kidney disease, 18
    laboratory evaluation of, 20–22
    management of, 22–26
    medicinal causes of, 19
    and natural medicines, 35
    and obesity, 12–13, 18–19
    and poststreptococcal acute
        glomerulonephritis, 71
    and renal failure, 6
    staging of, 13, 18

Hypertension in adolescents, 11–29

Hyperxaluria
    and urolithiasis, 97–98

Hypocitraturia
    and urolithiasis, 97

Hyponatremia
    in adolescent athletes, 113–114
    and antidiuretic hormone, 114

I

IBD. See Inflammatory bowel disease.

Idiopathic stones
    and urolithiasis, 104

Ifosfamide
    nephrotoxicity of, 139–141

Immune modulation
    and treatment of STDs, 58–60

Immunoglobulin A nephropathy, 50, 57
and glomerulonephritis, 72–74

Immunosuppression, 202–205

Implanon, 555

Inflammatory bowel disease
and contraception, 639

The Internet, 413–424
and academic information, 418–419
and access to information, 417–423
and adolescent online presence, 416–417
and digital-divide issues, 415
drinking portrayals on, 332
and eating disorders, 297–298
and illicit content, 275–276, 421–423
and influence on body image, 297–298
and information on social issues,
418–420
and parental filters, 424
and proanorexia web sites, 297–298
and probulimia web sites, 297–298
and sexual content, 275–276, 421–422
and social support and isolation,
415–416
and use among teenagers, 413–414
and violent content, 422–423

Intrauterine devices, 556–558, 592–594,
638–641
and contraception for chronically ill
adolescents, 638–641
copper versus progestin, 556
in developing countries, 650–651
as emergency contraception, 587–588,
592–594
Mirena, 556–558
ParaGard, 557

IUD. See Intrauterine devices.

J

Juxtaglomerular cell tumor, 128

K

Kidney biopsy
and nephrotic syndrome, 168–169
and STDs, 52–57

Kidney disease, 1–239
and biochemical parameters, 51
clinical and laboratory assessment for,
47–52
and creatinine clearance, 49–51
and cytomegalovirus, 54
and focal segmental glomerular sclerosis,
49–50, 53–55, 59
and glomerular filtration rate, 49–51

and hemolytic uremic syndrome,
49–50, 54
and hepatitis B virus, 45–46, 50, 54, 56,
58, 61
and hepatitis C virus, 45–46, 50, 54, 56,
58–59, 61
and HIV infection, 45–47, 49–51,
53–57, 59–62
and hypertension, 18
and immunoglobulin A nephropathy,
50, 57
and immunologic evaluation, 51–52
and immunologically mediated renal
lesions, 55–57
and membranoproliferative
glomerulonephritis, 50, 54, 56–57
and membranous nephropathy, 56
and non–immune-mediated renal
lesions, 53–55
and proteinuria, 48–49, 163–164
and radiologic studies, 51
and sexually transmitted diseases, 45–63
and systemic lupus erythematosus–like
variant, 49–50, 55–56
and treatment of STDs, 57–62
and tubulo-interstitial nephropathy,
49–50, 54–55
and urinalysis, 47–48
and viral assays for STDs, 47

Kidney failure. See Renal failure.

Kidney stones, 35, 87–107

Kidney transplantation, 61–62, 201–211
and acute rejection therapy, 206
and antibodies to interleukin-2
receptor, 203
and antilymphocyte globulin, 202–203
and antiproliferative agents, 205
and antithymocyte globulin, 202–203
and azathioprine, 204–205
and basiliximab, 203
and calcineurin inhibitors, 204–205
and cyclosporine, 203–204
and cytomegalovirus, 206, 208
and daclizumab, 203–204
and Epstein-Barr virus, 207–208
and growth and development, 209
and gynecologic issues, 209–210
and immunosuppression, 202–205
and induction therapy, 202
and infection, 206–207
and maintenance therapy, 204
and medication adherence, 208–209
and mycophenolate mofetil, 204–205
and OKT3 therapy, 202
and posttransplantation malignancy,
207–208
and quality of life, 210
and sirolimus, 205

and STDs, 61–62
and steroids, 204
and tacrolimus, 205

Kidney tumors, 121–142
    hereditary syndromes with, 128–131

Kidneys and sports, **111–119**

Klebsiella infection
    and urinary tract infections, 150, 153

L

Lactation
    and progestin-only contraception,
        558–559

Lactic acidosis
    and STDs, 60

Lea's shield, 510

Levonorgestrel, 521, 618, 620–622
    and emergency contraception, 588–593

M

Magazines
    drinking portrayals in, 332–333

Male antifertility herbs
    and *Anacardium occidentale*, 612
    and cotton plant, 611
    and herbal contraception, 611–612
    and nicotine, 611
    and papaya, 611
    and *Solanum xanthocarpum*, 612
    and thunder god vine, 611
    and *Tripterygium hypoglaucum*, 611

Male condoms, 489, 496–501

Male hormonal contraception, 628–629

MCD. See *Minimal change disease.*

Media
    drinking portrayals in, 327–333
    importance to teenagers, 272
    and sex education, 272–276
    and teenagers' perception of its influence,
        271–272

Media bias
    and media literacy, 466–467

Media literacy, 365, 463–479
    and adolescent smoking, 365
    effectiveness of, 476–478
    and media bias, 466–467
    and media violence, 470–471
    the need for, 465–469

and parental involvement, 477–478
popularity of, 471–472
principles of, 472–476
and product placement, 466

Media ratings for movies, music, video games,
    and television: a review of the research
    and recommendations for improvements,
    427–446

Media ratings systems
    and authority, 443
    consistency of, 435
    and construct validity, 437–438
    and content validity, 436–437
    and criterion validity, 438–439
    design of, 442–443
    and education, 443–444
    goals of, 433–439
    history and current configurations of,
        428–433
    and interrater reliability of, 434–435
    reliability and validity of, 433–434
    and research, 444
    and temporal stability, 435–436
    universal, 441–442

Media use among adolescents, 296–297

Media violence, 249–265
    amount of, 250–252
    and censorship, 263–264
    and desensitization in adolescents, 257,
        402–404, 476
    effects on adolescents, 255–257
    and fear in adolescents, 255–257
    and healthy media habits for
        families, 264
    and individual and social modifiers,
        259–260
    and media education, 262–263
    and media literacy, 470–471
    and media modifiers, 260–261
    and mitigation of effects, 261–264
    and parent education and monitoring,
        261–262
    and research validity, 252–255
    and role of media industry, 263–264
    and role of primary care provider,
        264–265
    and sports on television, 252
    and susceptibility among teens, 257–261
    and television news programs, 252,
        256–257
    and the V-chip, 262
    and video games, 252–254, 258, 261,
        264, 464, 467–471

Membranoproliferative glomerulonephritis, 50,
    54, 56–57, 68–69, 75–77, 167–168
    and nephrotic syndrome, 167–168

Membranous nephropathy, 56
and glomerulonephritis, 77–78

Menorrhagia
and oral contraceptive pills, 542

Menses
and progestin-only contraception, 543

Mental retardation
and contraception, 641–642

Metabolic abnormalities
and STDs, 60–61

Metabolic bone disease, 192–193

MI. See *Myocardial infarction.*

Microalbuminuria
and diabetic nephropathy, 176–177

Microbicides, 629, 632

Mifespristone
and emergency contraception, 588, 590,
592, 594

Minimal change disease
and nephrotic syndrome, 167–168

Mirena IUD, 556–558, 638–641

Mitral valve prolapse
and progestin-only contraception,
560–562

MMF. See *Mycophenolate mofetil.*

Movie ratings systems, 428–431

Movies
drinking portrayals in, 329–330
smoking in, 350–352

MTV
and effects of music videos on adolescent
health, 371–380, 383–384, 388
and sexual content, 278

Music lyrics
drinking portrayals in, 330–332

Music ratings system, 431

Music videos
adolescent audience for, 373
and attitudes toward violence, 383–384
and body image, 376–377, 385–386
drinking portrayals in, 330–332
and effect on teenage sexual activity, 278
and effects on adolescent health,
371–389
and gender roles, 376–377, 386–387
and health risks, 377–381
and influence on sexual attitudes,
384–385
and influence on substance use, 385

potential health benefits of, 387–388
protecting against the negative health
effects of, 387
and sexism, 376–377
and sexual content, 375–377
and sexual violence, 376–377, 386–387
and substance use portrayal, 375–376
and theories of media influence, 382
and viewer characteristics, 381–382
and violent content, 373–374, 376–377

MVP. See *Mitral valve prolapse.*

Mycophenolate mofetil
and kidney disease, 59, 74
and kidney transplantation, 204–205

Myocardial infarction
and oral contraceptive pills, 518

N

National Surveys of Family Growth, 486–487,
489–490

National Television Violence Study, 251, 257

National Youth Tobacco Survey, 346

Natural contraception, **603–616**
historical view, 604–606
and the Triobriand islanders, 604–605

Natural family planning, 603–606

Negative body image
exploring the results of, 292–294

Neisseria gonorrhea infection
and urinary tract infections, 154, 156

Nephrectomy
and hyperfiltration injury, 131–132
kidney function after, 131–135
and studies in children, 132
and Wilms tumor studies, 132–135

Nephrotic syndrome, 167–170
and ACE inhibitors, 170
and chlorambucil, 170
and corticosteroids, 169
and cyclophosphamide, 170
and cyclosporine, 170
and cytotoxic drugs, 169–170
and focal segmental glomerular sclerosis,
167–168
and immunosuppressive therapy,
169–170
and kidney biopsy, 168–169
and membranoproliferative
glomerulonephritis, 167–168
and minimal change disease, 167–168
and prednisone, 169
treatment of, 168–170

Nephrotoxicity
    and amphetamines, 40
    and Chinese herbs, 33–34
    and cocaine, 39
    and creatine, 34–35
    and drug abuse, 36–40
    and ecstasy, 40
    and heroin, 36–37, 39
    and inhalants, 39
    and natural medicines and dietary
        supplements, 32–38
    and nonsteroidal anti-inflammatory
        drugs, 32
    and over-the-counter analgesics, 31–32

Nephrotoxicity of over-the-counter analgesics,
    natural medicines, and illicit drugs,
    31–43

Neutrophilia
    and urinary tract infections, 153–154

NFSG. See *National Surveys of Family Growth.*

Nocturnal enuresis, 222–223

Non-Hodgkin's lymphoma, 124

Nonsteroidal anti-inflammatory drugs
    and acute renal failure, 115
    and nephrotoxicity, 32

Norgestimate, 521

Norplant, 555

NSAIDs. See *Nonsteroidal
anti-inflammatory drugs.*

O

Obesity
    and body image in the media, 292–293
    and hypertension, 12–13, 18–19
    and proteinuria, 166–167
    and school commercialism, 447–448,
        453–456

OCP. See *Oral contraceptive pills.*

Oral contraceptive pills, 489–491, 517–534
    advantages of, 523
    and adverse events, 522
    and cardiovascular disease, 546
    and cerebrovascular accidents, 518, 522
    and contraception for chronically ill
        adolescents, 636–642
    contraindications to, 522–523, 544
    and decreased acne, 523, 540–541
    and decreased benign breast disease,
        523, 541
    and decreased colorectal cancer, 540

    and decreased dysmenorrhea and
        menorrhagia, 523, 541–542
    and decreased ectopic pregnancy, 541
    and decreased endometrial cancer, 540
    and decreased fibroids, 542
    and decreased iron deficiency
        anemia, 542
    and decreased osteoporosis, 542
    and decreased ovarian cancers, 539
    and decreased ovarian cysts, 523, 540
    and decreased salpingitis, 541
    in developing countries, 651, 653
    disadvantages of, 523, 526
    efficacy of, 521–522
    as emergency contraception, 585–600
    and estrogen, 520
    formulation profiles of, 519
    and headaches, 546
    and improved symptoms in polycystic
        ovary syndrome, 542
    mechanism of action of, 519–520
    and myocardial infarction, 518
    noncontraceptive benefits of, 523,
        539–542, 627
    pharmacology of, 520–521
    and progestin, 521
    and stroke and transient ischemic
        attacks, 546
    and thromboembolism, 545–546
    and venous thromboembolism,
        518, 522

Osteoporosis
    and oral contraceptive pills, 542

Ovarian cancer
    and oral contraceptive pills, 539

Ovarian cysts
    and oral contraceptive pills, 540

Overview of contraception, **485–493**

Ovulation inhibition
    and asparagus, 609
    and the castor plant, 608–609
    and herbal contraception, 607–609
    and marshmallow plant, 609
    and Queen Anne's lace seeds, 607–608
    and the rivea plant, 608
    and stem bark extracts, 608
    and wild carrot, 607–608
    and wild yam, 609

Oxalate
    content in foods, 99

P

ParaGard IUD, 557

Paraneoplastic glomerulopathies, 137–138

Parenting style
and adolescent smoking, 356–358

Pauci-immune glomerulonephritis, 80

PCNL. See *Percutaneous nephrolithotomy.*

PD. See *Peritoneal dialysis.*

Pelvic inflammatory disease
and oral contraceptive pills, 541
and progestin-only contraception, 543

Pepsi Cola
and exclusive agreements with schools,
450–451, 453, 455

Percutaneous nephrolithotomy
and urolithiasis, 106

Peritoneal dialysis, 7

PID. See *Pelvic inflammatory disease.*

Polycystic ovary syndrome
and oral contraceptive pills, 542

Pornography
and changes in attitudes from exposure,
320–321
and effects in naturalistic settings,
321, 323
and exposure among teenagers, 317–318
individual differences in attraction to,
318–319
and the Internet, 275–276, 421–422
and link to rape, 321
sexual arousal to, 320
and sexually violent fantasies, 321–322

Pornography and teenagers: the importance of
individual differences, **315–326**

Poststreptococcal acute glomerulonephritis,
68–73
and hypertension, 71

Posttransplantation lymphoproliferative
disease, 207–208

Potassium disorders
and natural medicines, 37

Practical approaches to prescribing contraception in the office setting, **665–674**

Product placement
and media literacy, 466

Progestin
and emergency contraception, 587–593
and new developments in contraception,
622–624
and oral contraceptive pills, 521

Progestin-only contraception, 553–566
and cardiovascular disease, 547–548,
560–564
clinical indications for, 554, 558–565
contraindications to, 547–548
and deep vein thrombosis, 561–563
and diabetes, 564
as emergency contraception, 585–600
and gynecologic disorders, 560
and hepatobiliary disease, 565
and inherited hypercoagulable
disorders, 563
and lactation, 554, 558–559
and medical problems, 560–561
and mitral valve prolapse, 560–562
and neurologic conditions, 564
noncontraceptive benefits of, 543
and sickle cell disease, 564
and venous thromboembolism, 547–548

Progestin only contraceptives and their use in
adolescents: clinical options and medical
indications, **553–567**

Protein supplements
in adolescent athletes, 116

Proteinuria, 36, 48–49, 113, 163–167
in adolescent athletes, 113
and blood pressure, 167
and cardiovascular disease, 166
and diabetes, 166–167
and diet, 167
evaluating adolescents with, 166
and insulin deficiency, 166–167
and insulin-resistant conditions,
166–167
and kidney disease, 48–49, 163–164
and natural medicines, 36
and obesity, 166–167
testing for, 164–165
treatment of, 167

Proteus infection
and urinary tract infections, 150, 153
and urolithiasis, 103

PSAGN. See *Poststreptococcal
acute glomerulonephritis.*

PTLD. See *Posttransplantation
lymphoproliferative disease.*

Puberty
and diabetic nephropathy, 175–176

Pulmonary disease
and contraception, 639

Pyelonephritis, 149–158
treatment of, 158

Pyuria
and urinary tract infections, 153

R

Rap music lyrics
    and references to alcohol, 331–332

Rap music videos
    and influence on sexual behavior, 385
    and influence on violent behavior,
        383–384
    and portrayal of smoking, 376
    and violent content, 374

Rape
    and link to pornography, 321

Renal cancer, 121–142

Renal cell carcinoma, 123–124

Renal cystic disease
    acquired, 127

Renal disease
    and contraception, 638–639

Renal failure, 1–8
    diagnosis of, 4–5
    and dialysis, 6–7
    etiology of, 1–4
    and hemofiltration, 7
    and hyperkalemia, 5–6
    and hypertension, 6
    and obstruction, 4
    outcome of, 7–8
    therapy for, 5–7

Renal injury, 2–4

Renal lymphoma, 124–125

Renal manifestations of sexually transmitted
    diseases: sexually transmitted diseases
    and the kidney, **45–65**

Renal medullary carcinoma, 125–127

Renal perfusion
    inadequate, 2

Renal transplantation in adolescents, **201–214**

Renal tubular acidosis
    and STDs, 60

Reproductive health
    in developing countries, 649

S

Salpingitis
    and oral contraceptive pills, 541

School commercialism
    and Channel One, 448, 450
    and exclusive agreements, 449–457
    and soft drinks, 447–458

School commercialism and adolescent health,
    447–461

Seasonale, 527–528

Seizures
    and progestin-only contraception, 543

Sex education
    and the media, 272–276
    and sources of information, 272–273

Sex hormone binding globulin, 521

Sex in the media, 269–285
    and body image, 280–281, 289–307
    and contraceptive advertisements,
        278–281
    and eating disorders, 281–282, 293–296
    and effect on teenage sexual activity,
        276–277
    and MTV, 278
    and solutions for change, 282–285
    and solutions for health care
        providers, 283

Sexual content
    on the Internet, 275–276, 421–422
    in music videos, 375–377
    in television, 269–285

Sexually transmitted diseases, 45–63,
        151–155, 489, 492, 496, 498, 501–502,
        505–507, 646–650, 652, 654–660
    and adolescent surveillance, 62
    and angiotensin antagonists, 57–59
    and condoms, 496, 498, 501–502
    and the contraceptive sponge, 507
    in developing countries, 646–650, 652,
        654–660
    and dialysis, 60–61
    and HAART, 53, 56–58, 60–62
    and immune modulation, 58–60
    and kidney biopsy, 52–57
    and kidney disease, 45–63
    and kidney transplantation, 61–62
    and lactic acidosis, 60
    and metabolic abnormalities, 60–61
    and renal tubular acidosis, 60
    and spermicides, 505–506
    and treatment of kidney disease, 57–62
    and urinary tract infections, 151–155
    and viral assays, 47

Sickle cell disease
    and contraception, 640
    and progestin-only contraception, 564

SLE. See *Systemic lupus erythematosus.*

SmokeFreeMovies, 358–364

Smoking in movies: impact on adolescent
    smoking, **345–370**

Smoking initiation
heuristic model for the effect of media exposure on, 346–350

Snapple
and exclusive agreements with schools, 452

Social Learning Theory
and media influence, 382

Soft drinks
and exclusive agreements with schools, 449–457
and school commercialism, 447–458

Solitary kidney
in adolescent athletes, 116–117

Spermicidal agents, 503–506, 629, 632
advantages of, 504
and *Aloe barbadensis*, 610
and cotton plant, 610
disadvantages of, 504–505
efficacy of, 504
and herbal contraception, 610
and neem oil, 610
precautions for use of, 505–506
and prevention of STDs, 505–506
proper use of, 506
and *Sedum praealtum*, 610
and zinc acetate, 610

Spina bifida, 223

Sports
and acute renal failure, 114–115
and creatine use, 115
and end-stage renal disease, 117
and hematuria, 111–113
and hypertension, 117
and hyponatremia, 113–114
and kidney disease, 111–117
and protein supplements, 116
and proteinuria, 113
and solitary kidney, 116–117

Staphylococcus aureus infection
and urolithiasis, 103

Staphylococcus saprophyticus infection
and urinary tract infections, 150, 153

STDs. See *Sexually transmitted diseases.*

Stone disease, 218–220
surgical management of, 219–220

Systemic lupus erythematosus, 55–56, 68–69, 76, 80–81
and contraception, 641
and glomerulonephritis, 68–69, 76, 80–81

T

Telecommunications Act of 1996, 262

Television
and alcohol use in prime time, 328
drinking portrayals in, 327–329
and sexual content, 269–285
and sexually suggestive messages, 273
and violent content, 249–265

Television ratings system, 430, 432–433

TIN. See *Tubulo-interstitial nephropathy.*

TMP-SMX. See *Trimethoprim-sulfamethoxazole.*

Transdermal patch, 490, 528–532, 545, 624
advantages of, 531
and adverse events, 530–531
contraindications to, 531, 545
disadvantages of, 531–532
efficacy of, 530
and heart disease, 637–638
pharmacology of, 530

Trichomonas vaginalis infection
and urinary tract infections, 152

Trimethoprim-sulfamethoxazole
and urinary tract infections, 156–158

Tuberous sclerosis, 130–131

Tubulo-interstitial nephropathy, 49–50, 54–55

Tumor lysis syndrome, 135–137

U

Ureteropelvic junction obstruction, 216–218
surgical management of, 218

Uric acid
and urolithiasis, 98–101

Urinary calculi, 87–107

Urinary discoloration
causes of, 230

Urinary nitrites
and urinary tract infections, 153

Urinary stones, 87–107, 218–220
composition and structure of, 92

Urinary tract anomalies
delayed presentation of, 216–218

Urinary tract infections, 149–158
and bacteriuria, 153
and C-reactive protein, 153–154
causes of, 150
and colony counts, 153–154

diagnosis of, 154–156
differential diagnoses of, 151–152
and erythrocyte sedimentation rate,
    153–154
and *Escherichia coli*, 150, 153, 157
and hematuria, 153
and historical findings, 152
and laboratory findings, 153–154
and neutrophilia, 153–154
and pyuria, 153
and *Staphylococcus saprophyticus*,
    150, 153
and STDs, 151–155
treatment of, 156–158
and trimethoprim-sulfamethoxazole,
    156–158
and urinary nitrites, 153

Urinary tract infections among adolescents,
149–161

Urolithiasis, 87–107, 218–220
bacteriologic basis for, 88–89
clinical presentation of, 89–90
and cystinuria, 102–103
and 2,8-dihydroxyadenine calculi, 101
and extracorporeal shock wave
    lithotripsy, 106–107, 219
and hypercalciuria, 94–97
and hyperxaluria, 97–98
and hypocitraturia, 97
and idiopathic stones, 104
infection-related, 103–104
Laboratory studies for, 90–94
medical treatment of, 104–105
and percutaneous nephrolithotomy, 106
physical examination for, 90
physico-chemical basis for, 88–89
and *Proteus* infection, 103
radiologic evaluation of, 90–94
and *Staphylococcus aureus*
    infection, 103
surgical treatment of, 105–107
and uric acid, 98–101
and urinary excretion rates, 91–92
and xanthine stones, 101–102

Urolithiasis in adolescent children, **87–109**

UTI. See *Urinary tract infections.*

V

V-chip, 262, 305, 363–364
and media violence, 262
and smoking in movies, 363–364

Vaginal rings, 532–533, 545, 558, 624–625
advantages of, 533
and adverse events, 532–533

contraindications to, 533, 545
disadvantages of, 533
efficacy of, 532

Valenti, Jack
and the movie ratings system, 432, 434

Varicocele, 220–222

VATER syndrome, 216

Vending machines
in schools, 451–457

Venous thromboembolism
and oral contraceptive pills, 518, 522
and progestin-only contraception,
    547–548

Video games, **395–411**
and adolescent vulnerability, 398–399
and desensitization to violence,
    402–404, 476
and health benefits, 405
and health risks, 404–405
and playing time, 399–400
prosocial and educational, 397–398
and public policy issues, 406
ratings system for, 430–432
and recommendations for clinicians,
    407–408
and violent content, 395–397, 400–404,
    464, 467–471

Video killed the radio star: the effects of
music videos on adolescent health,
371–393

Violence
factors contributing to, 250
and the media, 249–265

Violent content
on the Internet, 422–423
in music videos, 373–374, 376–377
in television, 249–265
in video games, 395–397, 400–404,
    464, 467–471

Viral invasion
and mechanisms of local tissue injury,
    52–53

Voiding dysfunction, 222–224

Von Hippel-Lindau disease, 128–130

VTE. See *Venous thromboembolism.*

W

Weight gain
and depot medroxyprogesterone acetate,
    570–574

Wilms tumor, 122–123, 132–135
    and nephrectomy, 132–135

X

Xanthine stones
    and urolithiasis, 101–102

Y

Yasmin, 527

Youth Risk Behavior Survey, 383, 489–490

YRBS. See *Youth Risk Behavior Survey.*

Yuzpe regimen
    as emergency contraception,
        587–593, 628

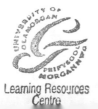

Changing Your Address?

Make sure your subscription changes too! When you notify us of your new address, you can help make our job easier by including an exact copy of your Clinics label number with your old address (see illustration below.) This number identifies you to our computer system and will speed the processing of your address change. Please be sure this label number accompanies your old address and your corrected address—you can send an old Clinics label with your number on it or just copy it exactly and send it to the address listed below.

We appreciate your help in our attempt to give you continuous coverage. Thank you.

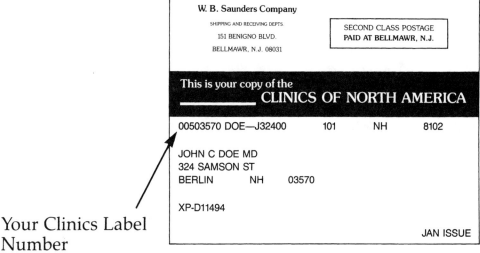

Your Clinics Label Number
Copy it exactly or send your label
along with your address to:
W.B. Saunders Company, Customer Service
Orlando, FL 32887-4800
Call Toll Free 1-800-654-2452

Please allow four to six weeks for delivery of new subscriptions and for processing address changes.